Cesarean Delivery: Its Impact on the Mother and Newborn, Part II

Guest Editors

LUCKY JAIN, MD, MBA
RONALD J. WAPNER, MD

CLINICS IN PERINATOLOGY

www.perinatology.theclinics.com

September 2008 • Volume 35 • Number 3

SAUNDERS an imprint of ELSEVIER, Inc.

W.B. SAUNDERS COMPANY
A Division of Elsevier Inc.

Elsevier, Inc. • 1600 John F. Kennedy Blvd. • Suite 1800 • Philadelphia, PA 19103-2899

http://www.theclinics.com

CLINICS IN PERINATOLOGY Volume 35, Number 3
September 2008 ISSN 0095-5108, ISBN-10: 1-4160-5800-1, ISBN-13: 978-1-4160-5800-7

Editor: Carla Holloway

Clinics in Perinatology (ISSN 0095-5108) is published in quarterly by Elsevier Inc., 360 Park Avenue South, New York, NY 10010-1710. Months of issue are March, June, September, and December. Business and Editorial offices: 1600 John F. Kennedy Blvd., Suite 1800, Philadelphia, PA 19103-2899. Customer Service Office: 6277 Sea Harbor Drive, Orlando, FL 32887-4800. Periodicals postage paid at New York, NY and additional mailing offices. Subscription prices are $197.00 per year(US individuals), $297.00 per year (US institutions), $232.00 per year (Canadian individuals), $369.00 per year (Canadian institutions), $268.00 per year (foreign individuals), $369.00 per year (foreign institutions) $95.00 per year (US students), and $131.00 per year (Canadian and foreign students). Foreign air speed delivery is included in all Clinics subscription prices. All prices are subject to change without notice. **POSTMASTER:** Send address changes to *Clinics in Perinatology*; Elsevier Periodicals Customer Service, 6277 Sea Harbor Drive, Orlando, FL 32887-4800. Customer Service: 1-800-654-2452 (US). From outside the United States, call 1-407-563-6020. Fax: 1-407-363-9661. E-mail: JournalsCustomerService-usa@elsevier.com.

Reprints. For copies of 100 or more, of articles in this publication, please contact the Commercial Reprints Department, Elsevier Inc., 360 Park Avenue South, New York, NY 10010-1710. Tel. (212) 633-3812; Fax: (212) 482-1935; email: reprints@elsevier.com.

Clinics in Perinatology is also pubilshed in Spanish by McGraw-Hill Interamericana Editores S.A., P.O. Box 5-237, 06500 Mexico D.F., Mexico.

Clinics in Perinatology is covered in *MEDLINE/PubMed (Index Medicus) Current Contents, Excepta Medica, BIOSIS and ISI/BIOMED.*

Printed in the United States of America.

GOAL STATEMENT
The goal of *Clinics in Perinatology* is to keep practicing neonatologists and maternal-fetal medicine specialists up to date with current clinical practice in perinatology by providing timely articles reviewing the state of the art in patient care.

ACCREDITATION
The *Clinics in Perinatology* is planned and implemented in accordance with the Essential Areas and Policies of the Accreditation Council for Continuing Medical Education (ACCME) through the joint sponsorship of the University of Virginia School of Medicine and Elsevier. The University of Virginia School of Medicine is accredited by the ACCME to provide continuing medical education for physicians.

The University of Virginia School of Medicine designates this educational activity for a maximum of 60 *AMA PRA Category 1 Credits™*. Physicians should only claim credit commensurate with the extent of their participation in the activity.

The American Medical Association has determined that physicians not licensed in the US who participate in this CME activity are eligible for *AMA PRA Category 1 Credits™*.

Credit can be earned by reading the text material, taking the CME examination online at http://www.theclinics.com/home/cme, and completing the evaluation. After taking the test, you will be required to review any and all incorrect answers. Following completion of the test and evaluation, your credit will be awarded and you may print your certificate.

FACULTY DISCLOSURE/CONFLICT OF INTEREST
The University of Virginia School of Medicine, as an ACCME accredited provider, endorses and strives to comply with the Accreditation Council for Continuing Medical Education (ACCME) Standards of Commercial Support, Commonwealth of Virginia statutes, University of Virginia policies and procedures, and associated federal and private regulations and guidelines on the need for disclosure and monitoring of proprietary and financial interests that may affect the scientific integrity and balance of content delivered in continuing medical education activities under our auspices.

The University of Virginia School of Medicine requires that all CME activities accredited through this institution be developed independently and be scientifically rigorous, balanced and objective in the presentation/discussion of its content, theories and practices.

All authors/editors participating in an accredited CME activity are expected to disclose to the readers relevant financial relationships with commercial entities occurring within the past 12 months (such as grants or research support, employee, consultant, stock holder, member of speakers bureau, etc.). The University of Virginia School of Medicine will employ appropriate mechanisms to resolve potential conflicts of interest to maintain the standards of fair and balanced education to the reader. Questions about specific strategies can be directed to the Office of Continuing Medical Education, University of Virginia School of Medicine, Charlottesville, Virginia.

The authors/editors listed below have identified no professional or financial affiliations for themselves or their spouse/partner:
Clarissa Bonanno, MD; Robert Boyle, MD (Test Author); Sreedhar Gaddipati, MD; Carla Holloway (Acquisitions Editor); Sameh M. Hussein, MD, MBBCH; Hassan M. Ibrahim, MD, MBBCH; Venkatakrishna Kakkilaya, MD, MBBS; Mark Bruce Landon, MD; Young MI Lee, MD; Melissa Mancuso, MD; Alan Mann, PhD; Russell Miller, MD; Fadi G. Mirza, MD; Janet Monge, PhD; Arun K. Pramanik, MD, MBBS; Charles R. Rardin, MD; Todd Rosen, MD; Dwight J. Rouse, MD, MSPH; Ronald J. Wapner, MD (Guest Editor); Kyle J. Wohlrab, MD; Blair J. Wylie, MD, MPH; and John A.F. Zupancic, MD, ScD.

The authors/editors listed below identified the following professional or financial affiliations for themselves or their spouse/partner:
Mary E. D'Alton, MD serves as a consultant for Artemis Health, Inc.
Richard Depp, MD serves on the Advisory Board and owns stock in US HealthConnect.
Lucky Jain, MD, MBA (Guest Editor) serves on the Speaker's bureau for IKARIA, and is an independent contractor for Schering Plough.
Stuart Weiner, MD serves on the Data Safety Monitoring Board for Repros Therapeutics, Inc.

Disclosure of Discussion of non-FDA approved uses for pharmaceutical products and/or medical devices:
The University of Virginia School of Medicine, as an ACCME provider, requires that all faculty presenters identify and disclose any "off label" uses for pharmaceutical and medical device products. The University of Virginia School of Medicine recommends that each physician fully review all the available data on new products or procedures prior to instituting them with patients.

TO ENROLL
To enroll in the Clinics in Perinatology Continuing Medical Education program, call customer service at 1-800-654-2452 or visit us online at www.theclinics.com/home/cme. The CME program is available to subscribers for an additional fee of $195.00

Contributors

GUEST EDITORS

LUCKY JAIN, MD, MBA
Richard W. Blumberg Professor; Executive Vice Chairman, Department of Pediatrics, Emory University School of Medicine, Atlanta, Georgia

RONALD J. WAPNER, MD
Professor of Obstetrics and Gynecology; Director of Maternal Fetal Medicine, Columbia University Medical Center, New York, New York

AUTHORS

CLARISSA BONANNO, MD
Fellow, Division of Maternal Fetal Medicine, Columbia Presbyterian Medical Center, New York, New York

MARY E. D'ALTON, MD
Professor and Chairman, Department of Obstetrics and Gynecology, Columbia University Medical Center, New York, New York

RICHARD DEPP, MD
Drexel University College of Medicine, Philadelphia, Pennsylvania

SREEDHAR GADDIPATI, MD
Assistant Clinical Professor, Division of Maternal Fetal Medicine, Columbia Presbyterian Medical Center, New York, New York

SAMEH HUSSEIN, MD, MBBCH
Assistant Professor of Pediatrics, Louisiana State University Health Sciences Center, Shreveport, Louisiana

HASSAN IBRAHIM, MD, MBBCH
Associate Professor of Pediatrics, Louisiana State University Health Sciences Center, Shreveport, Louisiana

VENKATAKRISHNA KAKKILAYA, MD, MBBS
Fellow of Neonatology, Louisiana State University Health Sciences Center, Shreveport, Louisiana

MARK B. LANDON, MD
Professor and Vice Chair, Department of Obstetrics and Gynecology; Director, Division of Maternal-Fetal Medicine, The Ohio State University College of Medicine, Columbus, Ohio

YOUNG MI LEE, MD
Assistant Professor, Division of Maternal-Fetal Medicine, Department of Obstetrics and Gynecology, Weill Cornell Medical College, New York, New York

MELISSA S. MANCUSO, MD
Division of Maternal Fetal Medicine, Department of Obstetrics and Gynecology, Center for Women's Reproductive Health, University of Alabama at Birmingham, Birmingham, Alabama

ALAN MANN, PhD
Professor of Anthropology, Department of Anthropology, Princeton University, Princeton, New Jersey

RUSSELL MILLER, MD
Division of Maternal Fetal Medicine, Department of Obstetrics and Gynecology, Columbia University Medical Center, New York, New York

FADI G. MIRZA, MD
Clinical Fellow, Division of Maternal-Fetal Medicine, Department of Obstetrics and Gynecology, Columbia University, New York, New York

JANET MONGE, PhD
Adjunct Professor of Anthropology; Acting Curator of Physical Anthropology, Department of Anthropology, University of Pennsylvania, University of Pennsylvania Museum of Archaeology and Anthropology, Philadelphia, Pennsylvania

ARUN K. PRAMANIK, MD, MBBS
Professor of Pediatrics, Louisiana State University Health Sciences Center, Shreveport, Louisiana

CHARLES R. RARDIN, MD
Assistant Professor, Alpert Medical School of Brown University, Division of Urogynecology, Women and Infants' Hospital of Rhode Island, Providence, Rhode Island

TODD ROSEN, MD
Assistant Clinical Professor of Obstetrics and Gynecology, Division of Maternal-Fetal Medicine, Department of Obstetrics and Gynecology, Columbia University, New York, New York

DWIGHT J. ROUSE, MD, MSPH
Division of Maternal Fetal Medicine, Department of Obstetrics and Gynecology, Center for Women's Reproductive Health, University of Alabama at Birmingham, Birmingham, Alabama

STUART WEINER, MD
Associate Professor, Department of Obstetrics and Gynecology; Director of Reproductive Imaging and Genetics, Division of Reproductive Imaging and Genetics, Maternal Fetal Medicine, Thomas Jefferson University and Hospital, Philadelphia, Pennsylvania

KYLE J. WOHLRAB, MD
Clinical Instructor, Alpert Medical School of Brown University, Division of Urogynecology, Women and Infants' Hospital of Rhode Island, Providence, Rhode Island

BLAIR J. WYLIE, MD, MPH
Instructor, Harvard Medical School, Division of Maternal-Fetal Medicine, Department of Obstetrics and Gynecology, Massachusetts General Hospital; Adjunct Assistant Professor of International Health, Center for International Health and Development, Boston University School of Public Health, Boston, Massachusetts

JOHN A.F. ZUPANCIC, MD, ScD
Assistant Professor of Pediatrics, Division of Newborn Medicine, Harvard Medical School; Department of Neonatology, Beth Israel Deaconess Medical Center, Boston, Massachusetts

Contents

Bipedalism and Parturition: an Evolutionary Imperative for Cesarean Delivery?   469

Stuart Weiner, Janet Monge, and Alan Mann

> Human biologic evolution involves a compromise between the physical adaptations for bipedalism with effects on birthing success and the much later increases in encephalization of our species. Much of what comes to define life history parameters like gestation length, and brain and birth weight in our species is best understood from this evolutionary perspective. Human populations have been dealing with the obstetric dilemma for many hundreds of thousands of years and modern biomedicine, using techniques like cesarean sections, has alleviated, but not eliminated, birthing as a "scar" of human evolution. If women begin to demand access to universal cesarean delivery, what will the outcome be for the future of human evolution? We can only speculate on the social, biologic, and demographic costs of this transition.

Cesarean Delivery for Abnormal Labor   479

Melissa S. Mancuso and Dwight J. Rouse

> Cesarean delivery is indicated at any stage in the labor process in the presence of nonreassuring fetal status or when conservative measures fail in the setting of abnormal labor. In the absence of maternal or fetal indications for expedited delivery, cesarean delivery is not indicated for latent phase disorders. When to intervene for protracted labor is arguable, but slow rates of labor progress are consistent with safe vaginal delivery. Cesarean delivery in the second stage should be avoided for at least 4 hours if there is progressive fetal descent.

Vaginal Birth After Cesarean Delivery   491

Mark B. Landon

> By 2004, only 9.2% of women in the United States with prior cesareans underwent a term of labor (TOL), although nearly two thirds of these women are actually candidates for a TOL. In this article, the author notes that the

principal risk associated with vaginal birth after cesarean delivery (VBAC)-TOL is uterine rupture, which can lead to perinatal death, fetal hypoxic brain injury, and hysterectomy. Risk factors for uterine rupture include number of prior cesareans, prior vaginal delivery, interdelivery interval, and uterine closure technique. The author concludes by noting that a pregnant woman with prior cesarean delivery is at risk for maternal and perinatal complications, whether undergoing TOL or choosing elective repeat operation. Complications of both procedures should be discussed and an attempt made to individualize the risk for uterine rupture and the likelihood of successful VBAC.

Mothers should be counseled that the most concerning risks related to maternal request cesarean delivery are neonatal respiratory morbidity and those that may affect the mother's future reproductive health, including life-threatening conditions, such as placenta accreta. The literature suggests that overall risks of maternal complications with cesarean delivery on maternal request are slightly lower than a trial of vaginal delivery and are primarily driven by the avoidance of unplanned or emergent cesarean deliveries and their associated increased rate of complications. When addressing risks and benefits with patients, there are three areas of importance. First, the risks for neonatal respiratory morbidity and abnormal placentation with future pregnancies should be emphasized. Secondly, there are many areas on which studies are lacking. Finally, numerous factors can alter the risks and benefits—such as culture, maternal obesity, and provider background—and should be acknowledged.

An unintended consequence of the rising cesarean section rate is abnormal placentation in subsequent pregnancies, leading to the clinical complications of placenta accreta and cesarean scar pregnancies. Both of these clinical entities are associated with high rates of maternal morbidity and mortality. This article reviews the potential mechanisms by which uterine scarring may lead to abnormal trophoblast invasion, the association of cesarean section with placenta accreta and scar pregnancies, current management, and suggestions for future research to reduce the incidence of these potentially devastating complications of pregnancy.

> Postpartum hemorrhage is an obstetric emergency that represents a major cause of maternal morbidity and mortality. With the recent rise in the cesarean delivery rate, prompt recognition and proper management at the time of cesarean delivery are becoming increasingly important for providers of obstetrics. Preparedness for hemorrhage can be achieved by recognition of prior risk factors and implementation of specific hemorrhage protocols. Medical and surgical therapies are available to treat obstetric hemorrhage after cesarean delivery.

> Despite advances in obstetric and neonatal care, the last several decades have not witnessed an improvement in the prediction or prevention of term cerebral palsy. Obstetric interventions such as electronic fetal heart rate monitoring and cesarean delivery, although biologically plausible as intervention strategies, do not improve perinatal outcomes in clinical practice. In reaction to mounting medicolegal pressure, obstetricians continue to increase the number of cesarean deliveries they perform as a form of defensive medicine, despite evidence that this practice is not associated with improved perinatal outcomes. The current standard for expeditious delivery in a case of potential fetal compromise is described by the "30-minute rule." However, obstetricians' determinations of the need for expedited delivery may be a preferable guide for appropriate delivery timing.

> Delay in cord clamping up to 30 to 40 seconds is feasible and should be practiced in preterm and term infants born by cesarean section. In term infants, this maneuver may decrease iron deficiency anemia at 6 months of age. Premature infants may have a higher blood volume and hematocrit initially requiring fewer transfusions. They also have a decreased incidence of intraventricular hemorrhage. The effect of compounding factors, such as maternal blood pressure, uterine contraction, medications, bleeding, and their effects on the infant's immediate and long-term outcome are unclear.

> Two trends are apparent regarding cesarean delivery in the developing world. In the least developed countries, access to the procedure remains limited at levels much less than 5% of all births. This limited access is linked with increases in maternal and neonatal mortality. Safety concerns are equally valid when more than half of women in certain socioeconomic strata are having surgical delivery, as is evident in the more advanced developing economies of Latin America and China. The optimal minimum and maximum cesarean delivery rates continue to be a matter of debate and may never be resolved; however, these two extremes of cesarean delivery use evident in the developing world deserve critical examination.

> Urinary and fecal incontinence have been linked to pregnancy and childbirth. This article reviews the rates of pelvic floor dysfunction following vaginal delivery and cesarean section as cited in short-term and long-term follow-up studies.

> Four million deliveries occur annually in the United States, and obstetric care has traditionally constituted a substantial portion of medical costs for young women, as well as being a major source of uncompensated care. The economic implications of a large shift in the mode of delivery are potentially important. This article reviews the relevant economic issues surrounding elective cesarean section and cesarean section at maternal request, summarizes the methodological quality and results of current literature on the topic, and presents recommendations for further study.

THE CLINICS ARE NOW AVAILABLE ONLINE!

Access your subscription at:
www.theclinics.com

Preface

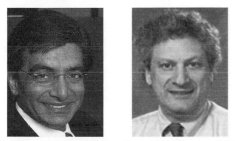

Lucky Jain, MD, MBA   Ronald J. Wapner, MD
Guest Editors

What kind of a delivery will our granddaughters have?

The rising frequency of cesarean sections has been well documented in both medical and lay literature. The excellent articles in the June 2008 issue of *Clinics in Perinatology* dedicated to cesarean delivery presented arguments for and against cesarean from a neonatal standpoint. This issue expands some of these concepts and adds additional information from the maternal and obstetrical standpoint.

Indeed, an in-depth study of the physiologic aspects of human parturition reveals many unanswered questions, and, as we begin to address these unknowns, we should remember that nothing is static, including human development. There is fascinating anthropological information that shows progressively increasing brain volume (hence, skull size) of the human fetus and concomitant changes in the pelvic anatomy as a result of bipedalism. These changes may have set up a natural conflict between vaginal birth and future generations.

There is evidence to show that cesarean births have improved outcomes in several high risk categories, such as breech presentation, very early gestations, and when there is clear evidence of fetal distress. However, these indications only represent a small portion of the increase in operative deliveries. Much of the increase comes from less certain speculation about the advantages. For example, it has been suggested that cesarean delivery will reduce the frequency of pelvic floor dysfunction and protect the infant against cerebral palsy. Yet, neither assertion has been scientifically validated.

As more patients are delivered by cesarean, new concerns have emerged about the short- and long-term risks and benefits to the mother. In particular, placenta accreta, uterine scar pregnancies and uterine rupture following attempted VBAC are seen with increasing regularity, putting the mother at risk in future pregnancies. The absence of clear evidence quantifying the short- and long-term risks and benefits of cesarean versus vaginal delivery has led to a conundrum, frequently confusing both patients and their health care providers. A panel of experts that met to discuss this issue under the auspices of the NICHD concluded that "virtually no studies exist on cesarean delivery on maternal request; given the limited data available, we cannot draw definitive conclusions about factors that might influence outcomes of planned cesarean delivery

Clin Perinatol 35 (2008) xv–xvi
doi:10.1016/j.clp.2008.08.001
0095-5108/08/$ – see front matter © 2008 Elsevier Inc. All rights reserved.

perinatology.theclinics.com

on maternal request versus planned vaginal delivery." This verdict notwithstanding, this decade will go down in history as the decade when "cesarean delivery on maternal request (CDMR)" became an official term in many developed nations. Despite this trend in developed nations, cesarean delivery remains unavailable in other parts of the world, even for the most urgent indications, reminding us of the inequities in health care that continue to exist today.

We are very grateful to Carla Holloway at Elsevier for her support with this project, and to all of our colleagues who have contributed to this issue. We hope that the two issues together will serve as a handy reference for a variety of topics related to cesarean birth. Meanwhile, the search for the ideal mode of delivery for our grandchildren, and their children, will continue!

Lucky Jain, MD, MBA
Department of Pediatrics
Emory University School of Medicine
2015 Uppergate Drive NE
Atlanta, GA 30322, USA

Ronald J. Wapner, MD
Columbia University Medical Center
622 W 168th Street
PH16-66
New York, NY 10032, USA

E-mail addresses:
ljain@emory.edu (L. Jain)
Rw2191@columbia.edu (R.J. Wapner)

Bipedalism and Parturition: an Evolutionary Imperative for Cesarean Delivery?

Stuart Weiner, MD[a],*, Janet Monge, PhD[b], Alan Mann, PhD[c]

KEYWORDS

• Evolution • Bipedalism • Partuition • Cesarean delivery

Bipedal locomotion is one of the major defining features of the human lineage and thus it has been involved in many subsequent changes that have occurred during the 6 to 8 million year course of human evolutionary history (based on femoral morphology of *Orrorin tugenensis*).[1] Once the changes in pelvic morphology are established for bipedal movement, increases in brain size are documented in our lineage, along with major changes in many life history variables, including many features associated with growth and development, both pre- and postnatally. Although these changes are precipitated through the processes associated with natural selection, this combination of changes produces a unique package of alterations in the reproductive biology and culture of humans. In the end, this parcel of evolutionary features results in a birth process that is, without medical intervention, painful and dangerous for mothers and their young. Abitbol[2] estimates that approximately 20% to 25% of human births, throughout the course of human evolutionary history, would end in maternal or fetal death. At the high end of this range, Keeler[3] has recorded a 30% maternal mortality, largely from obstructed labor, among the Kuna Indians of Panama as recently as the late twentieth century when parturition was managed with only traditional medicinal practices. For most of our evolutionary history, humans lived in small scale societies with only a few dozen reproductive-aged females. The loss of a significant portion of these

[a] Department of Obstetrics and Gynecology, Division of Reproductive Imaging and Genetics, Maternal Fetal Medicine, Thomas Jefferson University and Hospital, 834 Chestnut Street, Suite 400, Philadelphia, PA 19107, USA
[b] Department of Anthropology, University of Pennsylvania, University of Pennsylvania Museum of Archaeology and Anthropology, 3260 South Street, Philadelphia, PA 19104, USA
[c] Department of Anthropology, Princeton University, 123 Aaron Burr Hall, Princeton, NJ 08544, USA
* Corresponding author.
E-mail address: sweinermd@comcast.net (S. Weiner).

Clin Perinatol 35 (2008) 469–478
doi:10.1016/j.clp.2008.06.003
0095-5108/08/$ – see front matter © 2008 Elsevier Inc. All rights reserved.

females in childbirth would have had a profound effect on the society's demographic structure and, thus, ultimately on the evolutionary process.

Obligate human bipedalism (not to be confused with the occasional bipedalism displayed in many mammals, including other primates) is a unique form of locomotion generating a cascade of morphologic changes in the skeleton. Although other animals display varieties of habitual two-legged locomotion, human bipedalism is characterized by trunk uprightness and balance, along with the alternation of leg movements into swing and stance phases. To produce this type of motion, the human skeleton has gone through extensive modifications affecting literally every element. (For an excellent summary of these changes, see Aiello and Dean.)[4]

THEORIES ON THE ORIGIN OF BIPEDALISM

Various hypotheses on the origins of bipedalism and the locomotion of the last common ancestor of chimpanzees and humans have been proposed, beginning with Charles Darwin in 1871.[5] These hypotheses, although not all testable in the traditional sense, range from mechanical to behaviorally and culturally functional (reviewed in Richmond and colleagues).[6] On the most functional mechanical level, recent research by Sockel and colleagues[7] indicates that, compared with the quadrupedal locomotion of chimpanzees, human bipedalism is approximately 75% less costly in terms of energy consumption. Thus, it is possible that bipedalism evolved as a terrestrial adaptation that was an especially efficient form of locomotion. It is also possible that, although efficient in some ways, this locomotor system produced a much less speedy form of movement over a short distance but one which resulted in greater endurance. Under the right combination of environmental circumstances (eg, when the acquisition of sustenance or other resources required long distance movement), bipedalism, with its decreasing energetic cost, would be selected in favor of any form of quadrupedal movement.

Other hypotheses concentrate on the ensuing behavioral changes and emphasize one of the outcomes of bipedal locomotion: it frees the hands from the primary effort of locomotion. Initially, as suggested by Darwin,[5] most of these discussions concentrated on the use of tools as a primary component in understanding the origins of bipedalism. Although chimpanzees make, use, and even transport tools, and they are capable of bipedally locomoting over short distances, the requirements of rudimentary tool exploitation would thus not require consistent or obligate bipedality. Finally, in this context, present archaeologic evidence indicates that durable tools made from stone first appeared approximately 2.5 million years ago and therefore postdate the origin of bipedalism by several million years.

In 1981, Lovejoy[8] proposed a more holistic model for understanding not just the origins of bipedalism but also the host of characteristics that have come to define our evolutionary lineage. In this model, he proposed that bipedalism evolved as a way for male animals to carry food and provisions for female animals who were tending to the needs of the ever more immature young, another hallmark of our evolutionary lineage. Basic to this theory is that carrying, be it young altricial babies or food, was one of the major selective factors underlying the origin of this form of locomotion.

A previously dominant theory, the notion that bipedalism evolved as a protective device against predation,[9] has lost favor over the last several decades. In this model, bipedalism arose as a means to stand and look over the land to achieve a fuller view of the environment and thus to see potential predators before they could sense the presence of a vulnerable prey. The argument against this idea emphasized the possibility that in standing erect, not only would predators be seen more easily but potential prey would be viewed more easily by a predator. Further, although earlier models of the environment in which our lineage first evolved emphasized open grassland and savanna, recent data from various paleoenvironmental reconstructions now place these earliest bipedal ancestors in a more mosaic habitat that would have included grassland but also woodland and forest.

Finally, Wheeler[10,11] suggested that the advantage of bipedalism was as an adaptive protection against thermal stress. On the open savannah, quadrupedal animals expose more of their body surface area to the sun, whereas an erect biped would absorb 60% less heat at midday and be more fully exposed to any potential cooling breeze.

THE BIPEDAL PELVIS AND OTHER SKELETAL ADAPTATIONS

Although the reasons for the origins of bipedalism remain unknown, the modern human bipedal pelvis possesses anatomic features that came about as a result of this adaptation. These changes relate to unique aspects of the pelvis: those associated with weight bearing and balance on two, rather than four, legs and those related to muscle size and orientation, especially the relocation of the small gluteal muscles to a more lateral position, which modified their function to abduction **(Fig. 1)**.[12,13] These changes produced a vertically oriented pelvis, in contrast to the more horizontally oriented bones of the quadrupeds like those of the chimpanzee, with a birth canal constructed around three bony planes of fetal passage called

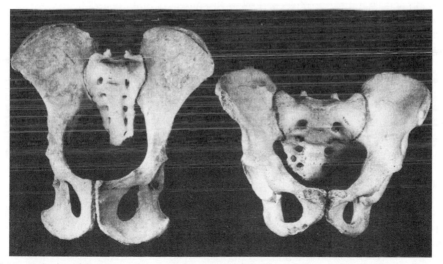

Fig. 1. Articulated human pelvis (*right*) compared to chimpanzee pelvis (*left*). The human pelvis is compressed with a greater girth in the horizontal plane in comparison to a chimpanzee, where the pelvis is narrow horizontally but very elongated in the vertical plane. This pelvic compression in humans, where the front and the back edge of the pelvis then come to sit on the same horizontal plane, is primarily responsible for the restrictive nature of the birth canal in humans. This bipedal change, in conjunction with the large brain size that comes to characterize our species, is the combination that produces the obstetrical dilemma in humans. The short and thickened iliac blades in the human pelvis are positioned laterally over hip joint sockets, thus repositioning G. *medius* and G. *minimus* and changing their function at the joint.

the inlet, midplane, and outlet. The bony structure of the birth canal in bipeds has become an elongated tube through which a fetus must navigate during the birth process. Also, to provide a wide base for upper body support and balance, the pelvis becomes overall ovoid in shape, flattened in the anterior-posterior direction relative to its width. In addition to the requirements associated with bipedalism and live birth, the pelvis must also support abdominal visceral weight and allow for the attachment on its superior surface of the major muscles of the trunk. These requirements led to changes in the pelvis that resulted in a relative narrowing from side to side at the midplane level relative to the inlet and outlet, resulting in a more complicated birth canal for the fetus to negotiate.[14]

Although the emphasis is primarily on the bony structures associated with bipedalism, it has become increasingly clear that major changes have occurred in the soft tissues associated with implantation and fetal growth requirements. Although humans share the characteristic hemochorial placenta of other higher primates, we are atypical in having a deeply invasive placenta of fetal trophoblast cells into maternal tissues and early implantation. These evolutionary distinctions from other primates may have occurred as a result of increased brain size and energetic requirements of the fetus, and as a means of filling the mechanical requirements of upright posture. As a result of these changes, humans are predisposed to preeclampsia and eclampsia,[15–17] perhaps, as suggested by the recent medical literature, when sufficient trophoblastic invasion fails to occur. However, as always, other explanations may exist because in some modern human cultures, such as in the Eskimos of Greenland and certain tribes in the South Pacific, toxemia does not occur.[18]

Thus, the bipedal pelvis serves two main functions: to produce efficient two-legged motion and, in female animals, to house the developing fetus and ultimately permit a successful birth outcome. It appears, however, that these two functions work in opposition to each other, with bipedal efficiency requiring a narrow, stable support and propulsion system but with birth requiring the opposite, a space as wide as possible within the internal dimensions of the bony birth canal. In modern humans, this development translates into a significant degree of sexual dimorphism in the pelvis, with women representing the greater compromise between these functions. Although we generally consider the normal female pelvis to conform to the general shape category termed "gynecoid" (one of the four general shape types that describe the internal dimensions of the pelvis), ample evidence shows that internal pelvic dimensions are a reflection of genetic and environmental processes[19] (for an excellent review, see).[20] It is also clear that no one shape best distinguishes male and female humans from each other.

Many other musculoskeletal features characterize the bipedal anatomic complex, beginning at the skull, with a centrally positioned foramen magnum, and moving distally to a host of alterations in the foot complex. A brief overview of these features is included in Harcourt-Smith.[21] One of the most important of these changes occurs in the production of the valgus angle of the femur to the knee joint and the production of the typical knocked-kneed appearance of humans. This necessary accommodation of the lower limbs to the requirements of bipedalism brings the lower limbs under the center of gravity, but the consequence is an unstable knee joint system (**Fig. 2**). Various changes occur in the foot, including the production of the three foot arches and changes in the orientation, function, and size of the hallux, with its new function of providing the final push off as a leg enters into its swing phase. The broad, laterally oriented shoulder girdle is characteristic of all the hominoids (apes and humans). This change within hominoid evolution has had important implications for the birthing process only in the human lineage after the evolution of the bipedal pelvis.

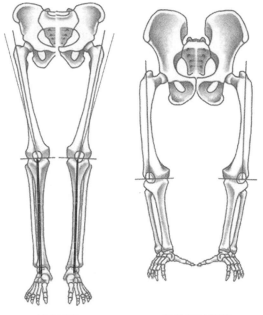

HUMAN   CHIMPANZEE

Fig. 2. Lower limbs of human and chimpanzee compared. There are immediately recogniz-able differences in lower limb anatomy between humans and our closest living relatives in virtually every bony element. In the pelvis, most importantly are the modifications made for weight bearing (eg, reduction in the overall vertical height of the pelvis) and for muscle position (most especially the reorientation of the small gluteal muscles). The valgus knee is also associated with bipedal locomotion. Notice that there is an accommodation at the knee to allow both an angulation of the femur from the hip to the knee but also to keep the knees parallel to the ground as well as maintaining their position directly under body weight. This angulation must by necessity be limited. *Black lines* how the position of the long axis of the major lower limb bones. *Red lines* show the effect of increasing diameter within the confines of the bony pelvis on the angulation of the femur from hip to knee. The lateral dimensions of the bony pelvis are limited by the degree of angulation possible of the femur from hip to knee while still maintaining the structural integrity of the knee joint. Given the incidence of knee injuries, especially in females with their wider hip joints, it is quiet possible we are at the limit of lateral hip expansion.

INCREASES IN BRAIN SIZE AND THE OBSTETRIC DILEMMA

Modern female humans and their infants experience a host of unique features associated with the birthing process. All of these together create a set of birthing features that ulti-mately result in what has been called the obstetric dilemma (but see also).[22] Rosenberg and Trevathan[16] summarize a unique set of features characterizing human birth:

1. Because of the tight fit of the fetus through the birth canal, the infant undergoes a series of rotations to maximize the success of the passage of the large infant head and shoulders into the changing dimensions of the maternal inlet, midplane, and outlet.
2. In general, the infant exits the birth canal in an occipital anterior position. In con-trast to other primates, where the neonate is born in a face-up position[23] allowing the mother to assist and lift her child to her nipples, the human infant exits

face downwards. Rosenberg and Travathan[16] argue that, as a result of this positioning, human childbirth requires assistance, a condition unknown in other mammals.

3. In human birth, the head and shoulders have a tight fit as the infant passes through the bony birth canal. Indeed, gestation length and the unique aspects of fetal growth and development appear to be dictated by the constraints produced during the birthing process.

4. Primate infants are generally considered precocial at birth; however, because of the constraints of the bony birth tube in humans (as described earlier) as a consequence of bipedalism, humans present newborns that are considered to show secondary altriciality. That is, in comparison with other primates, human babies are born with a much smaller proportion of adult brain size but a much larger body size. Secondary altriciality is really the production of a newborn at a stage of development that is similar to the prenatal periods of other primates and the human neonate is therefore more dependent on maternal feeding and care. Newborn human infants have often been called extrauterine fetuses.

5. Human infants are born immature in comparison with their primate cousins and to compensate for this immaturity, the postnatal period is characterized by a near doubling of brain size in the first year of postnatal growth.

When and why did this pattern of human birth occur in the human evolutionary record? The earliest members of our lineage, whose fossilized remains are complete enough that overall pelvis shape may be analyzed, are dated to approximately 3 million years ago and have been placed in the genus *Australopithecus* (AL288-1 [the Lucy pelvis], from Hadar, Ethiopia; Sts 14, from Sterkfontein, South Africa) (**Fig. 3**). This genus, limited to Africa, was the direct ancestor of the genus *Homo* and eventually of modern humans. The Australopithecines were fully and efficiently bipedal but possessed a brain size that was approximately one quarter the size of a modern human

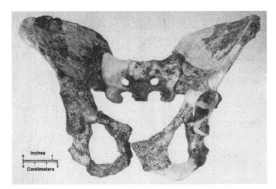

Fig. 3. The virtually complete pelvis of the australopithecine fossil from the site of Sterkfontein in South Africa (catalogue number Sts 14). Although the fossil is somewhat distorted—especially in the pubic rami on the right side (*left*), the sacrum contains only the first two of the total five elements, the basic restructuring associated with bipedalism is already in place in the 3 million-year-old specimen. There are some differences from the modern human pelvis shown in **Fig. 1**. For example, the ilia are more laterally positioned in Sts 14. Although there is some discussion as to the relevance manifest by these differences in the bipedal pattern of australopithecines and modern humans, virtually all researchers agree that the pattern of locomotion characterizing this extinct form was virtually identical to that used by modern humans.

brain (approximately 400 mL compared with modern human brains of between 1300 and 1400 mL). The reconstructed Australopithecine pelvis appears to possess a hyper-platypelloid shape with a markedly smaller anterior-posterior depth. Considering the limited fossil evidence and the lack of soft tissue, but also the bony tube shape of the pelvis and the small size of the adult and therefore fetus's brain at birth, general agreement does not exist as to whether or not early female humans would have experienced any of the problems associated with the obstetric dilemma.[24–26] Although it is generally agreed that the initial presentation of the infant during the birth process would have been to enter the inlet of the pelvis in the transverse plane, no agreement exists as to whether or not the infant would have undergone rotation as it moved into the midplane and outlet of the pelvis, although this mechanism is generally accepted in modern obstetrics.

The features of the obstetric dilemma probably first appeared sometime around the time of the origin of the genus *Homo*, approximately 2.5 to 2 million years ago, when brain size almost tripled, body size increased dramatically, and the pelvis began to expand in an anterior-posterior dimension and take on a more modern human shape. Although no general agreement exists as to what part of the package of the obstetric set of characteristics had evolved by this time, the combination of alterations in pelvic morphology with enlarging brains indicates that the pattern of human childbirth had begun to emerge.[27–30] By 300,000 years ago, brain size and pelvic morphology were essentially identical to that of modern humans and the assumption is that the birth mechanism had also taken on its modern form.[16]

One grouping of fossil hominids has taken on a special significance in human evolutionary studies associated with the obstetric dilemma. The Neandertals, broadly ranging in time from about 150,000 to 30,000 years ago, and inhabiting many areas in Europe and the Middle East, have a unique elongated pubic bone morphology along with what many researchers consider a larger brain size (an average of approximately 1500 mL) than what is generally considered the average of modern humans. Using this combination of features, Trinkaus[31] hypothesized that Neandertal gestation was 12 to 14 months in duration. Although many interesting discussions ensued from this provocative hypothesis, especially by Rosenberg,[32] this issue became part of a broader discussion surrounding the complex relationship of maternal body and pelvic dimensions to fetal dimensions. Although it is accepted that it is primarily maternal height, then weight, that are directly related to fetal birth weight,[33,34] with the body mass index being the most influential overall, the relative proportions of maternal pelvic dimensions and fetal head size are still uncertain.[35]

Finally, what is most remarkable in the evolutionary history of humans is the obvious strong selective pressure for increases in brain size. The obstetric dilemma has at its essential core the necessity for large brains as part of the package of emerging humanness. Selection was apparently so strong for the ensuing complex behaviors that came to characterize humans that it more than compensates for the difficulties associated with the birthing process. Associated with these complex behaviors is the necessity for the birth event and the rearing of newborns to take on a social context, perhaps beginning with obligate midwifery and pair bonding. These social institutions were made necessary by the evolution of the enlarging brain and the limitations imposed on the birth process by the needs of a bipedal pelvis.

THE CULTURAL IMPERATIVE FOR CESAREAN DELIVERY

At about the time of the Industrial Revolution, medical attention to childbirth began to transfer away from traditional midwifery to obstetric physician attendance. The use of ancient Chinese/Japanese, then British, instruments to assist difficult deliveries was followed by the use of the obstetric forceps and attention given to the notion that the fetus had its own environment, important circulatory physiology, and demands. Although the concept of cesarean delivery had been documented (and even mandated when maternal death occurred) since Roman times, this procedure was not deemed safe and life saving until the advent of antisepsis, antibiotics, and blood transfusions in the early twentieth century. Since then, an increasing balanced emphasis on saving the mother and infant has led to a progressive interest in the redemptive value of cesarean delivery.

Through the latter half of the twentieth century, concern for the delivery of a "healthy" baby has led to further technologic advances. With the advent of electronic fetal heart rate monitoring and conduction (especially epidural) anesthesia, and a progressive decline in instrumental or operative delivery (viewed as too traumatic), a cultural change has occurred in what is viewed as a "normal" delivery. Additionally, increasing concerns about the causes of cerebral palsy and the medicolegal defense of same, more recent desires to preserve maternal pelvic floor musculature (for sexual and urinary/anal continence) and to address celebrity and workforce issues of the increasingly elderly gravida, and the scheduling and safety of delivery, have all led to a dramatic increase in the rate of cesarean delivery. Although the United States rate has recently surpassed 30%, birth statistics in regions of China and Brazil reveal a cesarean delivery rate of 60% or higher. Simultaneously, the ethical principles of maternal autonomy, physician beneficence, and societal justification of the allocation of medical care resources have all come to the forefront in medical decision making. Plante[36] has thoroughly reviewed these influences and the costs to the patient and society of the increasing cesarean delivery rate and the recent rise in the gravida's request for "cesarean on demand." She has aptly elucidated the benefits of cesarean delivery on maternal request against the financial costs to society, and the medical risks for increased maternal morbidities for current and especially future pregnancies, including the risks for abnormal placentation, uterine rupture, and visceral organ injury with future child bearing.

CONCLUSION: WHENCE HUMAN CHILD BEARING AND WHAT ARE THE CONSEQUENCES?

The fossil record of human evolution suggests that vaginal birth is indeed dangerous for women of child-bearing age and their offspring. Encephalization can be documented using the fossil record and it is clear that over the last 2 million years, this process has come at a dramatic cost to our species when viewed in concert with the evidence of the early development in our lineage of obligate bipedal movement. What has also become clear is that it is human to involve social and cultural agencies to alleviate some of the biologic cost of this combination. The origin lies first with the need for aid during childbirth, met by enlisting the help of relatives and friends as midwives. Later, the medicalization of childbirth and improvements in the technology associated with childbirth, although only evident for the past 200 years, a mere blip in the face of 6 million years of the fossil record, clearly mandate the least mortality risk for human parturition, despite possible higher societal costs.

How far will this trend go? What will be the consequences of universal cesarean delivery? Can we predict the possible effects on humans of almost total disassociation of childbirth from vaginal delivery? If the trends thus far are any indication, it seems clear that women with access to medical care and with adequate financial support opt for cesarean delivery more often than is absolutely imperative based purely on the mechanics of delivery through the hard tissues of the pelvic birth tube. Will the end result be a change in the overall balance between fetal brain size and the biomechanical properties of the pelvis associated with birth and with the limitations imposed by successful bipedal functionality? If yes, it is impossible to predict the direction or extent of that change.

SUMMARY

Human biologic evolution involves a compromise between the physical adaptations for bipedalism with effects on birthing success and the much later increases in encephalization of our species. Much of what comes to define life history parameters like gestation length and brain and birth weight in our species is best understood from this evolutionary perspective. Human populations have been dealing with the obstetric dilemma for many hundreds of thousands of years and modern biomedicine, using techniques like cesarean sections, has alleviated, but not eliminated, birthing as a "scar" of human evolution. If women begin to demand access to universal cesarean delivery, what will the outcome be for the future of human evolution? We can only speculate on the social, biologic, and demographic costs of this transition.

REFERENCES

1. Richmond B, Jungers WL. *Orrorin tugenensis* femoral morphology and the evolution of hominin bipedalism. Science 2008;319:1662–5.
2. Abitbol MM. Birth and human evolution: anatomical and obstetrical mechanics in primates. Westport (CT): Bergin & Garvey; 1996.
3. Keeler CE. Land of the moon-children: the primitive san blas culture in flux. Athens (GA): University of Georgia Press; 1956.
4. Aiello L, Dean C. An introduction to human evolutionary anatomy. New York: Academic Press; 1990.
5. Darwin C. The decent of man, and selection in relation to sex. London: John Murray; 1871.
6. Richmond B, Begun D, Strait D. Origin of human bipedalism: the knuckle-walking hypothesis revisited. Yearb Phys Anthropol 2001;44:70–105.
7. Sockol MD, Raichlen DA, Pontzer H. Chimpanzee locomotor energetics and the origin of human bipedalism. Proc Natl Acad Sci U S A 2007;104:12265–9.
8. Lovejoy CO. The origin of man. Science 1981;211:341–50.
9. Dart R. *Australopithecus africanus*: the ape-man of South Africa. Nature 1925; 115:195–7.
10. Wheeler PE. The evolution of bipedality and loss of functional body hair in homininds. J Hum Evol 1984;13:91–8.
11. Wheeler PE. The influence of bipedalism on the energy and water budgets of early hominids. J Hum Evol 1991;21:117–36.
12. Lovejoy CO. The gait of Australopithecines. Yearb Phys Anthropol 1974;17: 147–61.
13. Lovejoy CO. Evolution of human walking. Sci Am 1988;259:118–25.
14. Rosenberg KR, Trevathan WR. The evolution of human birth. Sci Am 2001;415: 76–81.
15. Rockwell LC, Vargas E, Moore LG. Human physiological adaptation to pregnancy: inter- and intraspecific perspectives. Am J Hum Biol 2003;15:330–41.
16. Rosenberg KR, Trevathan WR. An anthropological perspective on the evolutionary context of preeclampsia in humans. J Reprod Immunol 2007;76:91–7.
17. Martin RD. Human reproduction: a comparative background for medical hypotheses. J Reprod Immunol 2003;59:111–35.

18. Moore ML. The importance of culture in childbearing. J Obstet Gynecol Neonatal Nurs 1972;1:29–32.
19. Arbitol M. Obstetrics and posture in pelvic anatomy. J Hum Evol 1987;16:243–55.
20. DelPrete HA. Secular changes in the morphology of the modern human pelvis and the implications for human evolution. Ph.D. Dissertation, Rutgers University, Department of Anthropology. 2006.
21. Harcourt-Smith WEH. The origins of bipedal locomotion. In: Henke W, Tattersall I, editors, Handbook of paleoanthropology, vol. 3. New York: Springer; 2007. p. 1484–518.
22. Walrath D. Rethinking pelvic typologies and the human birth mechanism. Curr Anthropol 2003;44:5–31.
23. Trevathan WR. The evolution of bipedalism and assisted birth. Med Anthropol Q 1996;10:287–98.
24. Rosenberg KR. The evolution of modern human childbirth. Yearb Phys Anthropol 1992;35:89–124.
25. Tague R, Lovejoy CO. The obstetrical pelvis of A.L. 288-1 (Lucy). J Hum Evol 1986;15:237–55.
26. Berge C, Orban-Segebarth R, Schmid P. Obstetrical interpretation of the australopithecine pelvic cavity. J Hum Evol 1984;13:573–87.
27. Martin RD. Human brain evolution in an ecological context. 52nd James Arthur lecture on the evolution of the human brain. New York: American Museum of Natural History; 1983.
28. Walker A, Ruff CB. The reconstruction of the pelvis. In: Walker A, Leakey REF, editors. The nariokotome Homo erectus skeleton. Cambridge (MA): Harvard University Press; 1993. p. 221–33.
29. Ruff CB. Biomechanics of the hip and birth in early Homo. Am J Phys Anthropol 1995;98:527–74.
30. Wittman AB, Wall LL. The evolutionary origins of obstructed labor: bipedalism, encephalization, and the human obstetrical dilemma. Obstet Gynecol Surv 2007;62:739–48.
31. Trinkaus E. Neandertal pubic morphology and gestation length. Curr Anthropol 1984;25:509–14.
32. Rosenberg KR. The functional significance of Neandertal pubic length. Curr Anthropol 1988;29:595–617.
33. Bhattacharya S, Campbell DM, Liston WA, et al. Effect of body mass index on pregnancy outcomes in nulliparous women delivering singleton babies. BMC Public Health 2007;7:168–76.
34. Guihard-Costa A-M, Papiernik E, Kolb S. Maternal predictors of subcutaneous fat in the term newborn. Acta Paediatr 2004;93:346–9.
35. Allbrook D, Sibthorpe EM. A study of pelvic dimensions related to infant size in the Ganda of East Africa. S Afr J Med Sci 1961;26:73–83.
36. Plante LA. Public health implications of cesarean on demand. Obstet Gynecol Surv 2006;61:807–15.

Cesarean Delivery for Abnormal Labor

Melissa S. Mancuso, MD*, Dwight J. Rouse, MD, MSPH

KEYWORDS

- Cesarean section • Abnormal labor • Failure to progress
- Dystocia • Cephalopelvic disproportion

Labor is the physiologic process by which the fetus is expelled from the uterus.[1] By definition, labor refers to regular uterine contractions that result in progressive dilation and effacement of the cervix and lead to descent and expulsion of the fetus. In a general sense, abnormal labor refers to a process that deviates from what most women undergoing spontaneous vaginal delivery experience. Abnormal labor affects nearly 20% of parturients and is the most common indication for primary cesarean delivery.[2] Such abnormalities have been described as dystocia, dysfunctional labor, failure to progress, and failure to descend. Because many repeat cesarean deliveries are performed because of a prior cesarean for dystocia, an estimated 60% of all cesarean deliveries are attributable to abnormal labor.[3]

When to intervene with a cesarean delivery for abnormal labor progress is controversial. It is clear that the difference between what is considered normal and sufficiently abnormal to warrant operative intervention remains a gray area, and much room for clinical judgment exists. That said, there is an evidence base on which to make the necessary judgments.

In 1955, Friedman published a landmark study from which the eponymous "Friedman curve" was derived. The Friedman curve depicts what has long been recognized as the normal progression of labor. From that work came the establishment of a series of definitions of protraction and arrest disorders of labor. These definitions achieved widespread acceptance. More recent data suggest that the traditionally accepted definitions of normal and abnormal labor progress may be less relevant to the contemporary gravida, as both she and labor management and practice have evolved.

Friedman's original work focused on women who presented in spontaneous labor. The majority of those women did not have regional anesthesia, were not induced, and infrequently received oxytocin. Many had an operative vaginal delivery. In

Division of Maternal Fetal Medicine, Department of Obstetrics and Gynecology, Center for Women's Reproductive Health, University of Alabama at Birmingham, 619 19th Street South, Old Hillman Building Room 446, Birmingham, AL 35249-7333, USA
* Corresponding author.
E-mail address: mmancuso@uab.edu (M.S. Mancuso).

Clin Perinatol 35 (2008) 479–490
doi:10.1016/j.clp.2008.06.004
0095-5108/08/$ – see front matter © 2008 Elsevier Inc. All rights reserved.
perinatology.theclinics.com

contemporary practice, labor induction is a common practice, and oxytocin use in the active phase is widespread. Most nulliparas who labor do so with regional analgesia. Vaginal breech and midforceps deliveries are rarely performed. Women are heavier, and their increased soft tissue mass may be an impediment to vaginal birth.

This article focuses on the available, contemporary literature and provides definitions of various labor abnormalities that are sufficient to warrant cesarean delivery. For the purposes of this article, the focus is on nulliparous women giving birth to a singleton fetus in vertex presentation. These women are the focus because abnormal labor is the most common indication for primary cesarean delivery, and the rate of cesarean delivery among nulliparas is the principal determinant of the overall cesarean delivery rate. Cesarean delivery for nonreassuring fetal status is beyond the scope of this article.

NORMAL LABOR

The genius of Friedman was to graph cervical dilatation against time. He then separated labor into three functional divisions: the preparatory division, the dilatational division, and the pelvic division.[4] The preparatory division, or latent phase, is the time in which cervical stromal and connective tissue changes are taking place without marked dilation of the cervix. This "cervical ripening" can occur in the presence or absence of regular contractions. The dilatational phase, or active phase, is the time in which dilation of the cervix occurs at its maximum rate of change. Friedman subdivided the active phase into the acceleration phase, or phase of maximum slope, and the deceleration phase, during which the cervical dilation continues—but at a slower pace—until full dilation. The pelvic division, or second stage of labor, is the time from complete cervical dilation to delivery of the infant. Within these divisions are the more commonly referred to "stages of labor." The first stage of labor is the time from onset of labor to complete cervical dilatation. The preparatory division and dilatational division together make up the first stage of labor. The second stage is the time from complete cervical dilatation to expulsion of the fetus (ie, Friedman's pelvic division). The third stage of labor is the time from expulsion of the fetus to expulsion of the placenta.

Friedman's establishment of "mean" labor curves defined the limits of normal labor on the basis of statistical deviations from the mean cervical-dilatation-time curve in women who delivered vaginally.[5] As such, these labor curves can aid in determining which parturients deviate from the norm and may require intervention.

CLASSIFICATION AND DIAGNOSIS OF LABOR ABNORMALITIES

Labor abnormalities are best categorized as protraction disorders or arrest disorders. Protraction involves slower progress than normal. Arrest disorders involve complete cessation of progress. Protraction and arrest disorders can occur in the first and second stages of labor.

LATENT PHASE DISORDERS

Latent labor as defined by Friedman is the point at which regular uterine contractions are perceived. It is generally thought that the latent phase has ended when cervical dilatation is between 3 and 4 cm.[3] Friedman reported that the mean duration of latent labor is 6.4 hours for nulliparas and 4.8 hours for multiparas.[5] In a more recent cohort, mean latent phase for nulliparas who delivered vaginally was reported to be 10.8 hours.[6]

Abnormalities of latent phase labor occur in 3.6% of nulliparous women.[7] Arrest of the latent phase implies that labor has not begun. Protracted latent phase occurs when latent labor lasts longer than 20 hours in nulliparas and 14 hours in multiparas.[7] Latent phase labor is highly variable and for some women is quite long. In these cases, expectant management is preferred. Therapeutic rest also may be prescribed using a pharmacologic agent, such as morphine, especially those women in whom contractions are painful. Early amniotomy is not recommended in nulliparas with protracted latent phase because it may increase the risk of infectious morbidity secondary to prolonged rupture of membranes. In the absence of other maternal or fetal indications for expedited delivery, cesarean delivery is not indicated for abnormalities of the latent phase.

FAILED INDUCTION

Arrest of the latent phase simply implies that labor has not begun. In cases in which delivery is indicated, augmentation or induction of labor may be appropriate. Compared with spontaneous labor, induced labor is longer and has increased risk of infection and cesarean delivery. Those risks are influenced by the status of the cervix at the time of induction. Induction of labor with an unfavorable cervix (Bishop score $\leq$ 6) increases the length of the latent phase.[8]

The rate of labor induction in the United States increased from 9.5% in 1990 to 21.2% in 2004 and continues to rise.[9] Despite the frequency of labor induction, consensus criteria for failed labor induction have not been established. Current national guidelines for the performance of cesarean delivery are directed only at women in active phase labor. The increasing prevalence of labor induction and the lack of an accepted definition for failed induction almost certainly contribute to unnecessary cesarean deliveries. An evidence-based definition for induction of labor failure should maximize the number of women progressing to the active phase and ultimately delivering vaginally while maintaining a low risk of maternal and neonatal adverse outcomes.[10] Surprisingly, only three studies have evaluated criteria for failed labor induction.

In the first study, Rouse and colleagues in 2000[11] developed and prospectively instituted a protocol that defined failed labor induction using two criteria: duration of ruptured membranes after initiation of oxytocin and lack of progression into the active phase of labor. They tested the safety and efficacy of that protocol in 509 women, 360 (71%) of whom were nulliparous. If the fetal heart rate pattern was reassuring, cesarean delivery before the active phase of labor (defined as cervical dilation of at least 4 cm and 90% effacement or 5 cm of cervical dilation) was not permitted for nonprogressive labor before oxytocin had been administered for at least 12 hours *after* ruptured membranes. Once in the active phase, labors were managed according to the previously published active phase labor management protocol.

Twenty-five percent of nulliparas and 9% of multiparas underwent cesarean delivery. In nulliparas, the median interval from oxytocin initiation to rupture of membranes in women who began induction with intact membranes was 6.3 hours, and the median induction-to-delivery interval was 14.2 hours. In nulliparas who began induction with ruptured membranes, the median induction-to-delivery interval was 9.2 hours. After 6 hours of oxytocin with ruptured membranes, 14% ($n = 51$) of nulliparas were still in the latent phase. Of those 51 women, 39% ($n = 20$) achieved successful vaginal delivery. Seven percent ($n = 25$) remained in latent phase after 9 hours; their vaginal delivery rate was 28%. Only 4% ($n = 15$) remained in the latent phase after 12 hours, and 13% of those women achieved vaginal delivery. Nulliparas in the latent phase 6, 9, and

12 hours after oxytocin initiation and ruptured membranes had higher rates of infectious morbidity (chorioamnionitis and endometritis) than women who progressed to the active phase or delivered at those stages, although the difference was statistically significant only for endometritis. The intervals were significantly shorter in parous women. When compared with nulliparas, parous women were less likely to remain in the latent phase after 6 hours of oxytocin and ruptured membranes (14% versus 3%, respectively). Of the five parous women still in latent phase after 6 hours, two were still in the latent phase at 9 hours and none was in the latent phase at 12 hours. All of these women achieved vaginal delivery.

None of the women in this cohort suffered severe morbidity. No maternal outcomes—except for cesarean delivery and infectious morbidity—among nulliparas correlated with length of the latent phase, including postpartum hemorrhage, blood transfusion, wound infection, and length of stay. The rate of serious neonatal morbidity was unrelated to latent phase duration. Twelve infants had serious neonatal morbidities. Ten of these 12 infants were born to mothers who had progressed to the active phase or were delivered after 6 hours of oxytocin and ruptured membranes. Only 1 of these 12 infants was born to a nullipara who was in the latent phase after 6 hours. Rates of less severe neonatal morbidities, such as treatment with antibiotics, shoulder dystocia, oxygen requirement, and length of stay, did not correlate with latent phase duration.

This study demonstrated that by requiring a minimum of 12 hours of oxytocin after membrane rupture before failed labor induction could be diagnosed, a substantial proportion of nulliparas who had slow progression to the active phase could achieve safe vaginal delivery.[11] This investigation was an important initial attempt at standardizing the definition of failed labor induction and did so based on reproducible and pertinent clinical parameters.

Simon and Grobman[12] were the second to address this subject when in 2005 they evaluated 400 nulliparous women who had undergone induction of labor. Their objective was to correlate the length of the latent phase with rates of vaginal delivery and maternal and neonatal adverse outcomes. In this cohort, the median time from initiation of oxytocin to artificial rupture of membranes was 1 hour. The median interval from amniotomy until active labor was 6.4 hours and from amniotomy to delivery was 10.9 hours. Two hundred thirty-six (59%) women achieved spontaneous vaginal delivery, 54 (15%) had operative vaginal deliveries, and 109 (26%) underwent cesarean delivery. The risk of cesarean delivery increased with increasing duration of the latent phase; however, one third of women still in the latent phase even after 18 hours achieved safe vaginal delivery. Chorioamnionitis and postpartum hemorrhage increased with increasing duration of the latent phase; however, this did not translate into increased transfusion rates or increased length of stay. Neonatal morbidities did not increase with increasing duration of the latent phase. Simon and Grobman[12] demonstrated that most women who remained in latent labor despite ruptured membranes and oxytocin at 12 hours achieved vaginal delivery.

In 2007, Blackwell and colleagues[6] were the third group to evaluate the relationship between duration of labor induction and vaginal delivery in nulliparous women by studying singleton pregnancies 37 weeks' gestation or more. During the 1-year study period, 340 women met criteria for entry into the study; 305 of these women reached active phase labor. Despite the fact that half of these women had an unfavorable cervix at induction initiation (modified Bishop score < 2), 75% achieved vaginal delivery.

Most women (69.3%) delivered within 24 hours, and 19 women remained undelivered at 48 hours. The duration of latent phase labor (defined as time first cervical ripening agent was given until time cervical dilation reached 4 cm) for women who achieved vaginal delivery at the 50th, 90th, and 95th percentiles was 10.8, 26.6, and 33.3 hours, respectively. The respective durations of active phase labor were 5.6, 11.2, and 13.6 hours. There was no relationship between greater induction to delivery time and endometritis, postpartum hemorrhage, fetal acidemia, or admission to neonatal intensive care unit. Of note, 40.6% of these women who achieved vaginal delivery had cervical dilation less than 1 cm/h in the active phase.[6]

Based on the available contemporary literature, it is clear that cesarean delivery should be performed infrequently for nonprogressive labor in the latent phase. In the aforementioned studies, only 4%[11], 10%[12], and 2%[6] of nulliparas underwent cesarean delivery before exiting the latent phase. In all three studies, neonatal outcomes were unrelated to latent phase duration. The only maternal morbidities that correlated with increasing latent phase duration were chorioamnionitis and postpartum hemorrhage (but not transfusion, hysterectomy, or prolonged hospital stay).

The duration of oxytocin administration after membrane rupture is a reproducible metric that can be used to judge the adequacy of attempted induction and define a "failed induction." The previously mentioned studies support that this duration should be at least 12 hours and that abnormal latent labor sufficient to warrant cesarean delivery should be defined as failure to reach a cervical dilation of 4 cm with 90% effacement or 5 cm dilation regardless of effacement after a minimum of 12 hours of oxytocin after membrane rupture. Prior to this, in the absence of another indication for delivery, cesarean delivery should not be performed. If the fetal heart rate pattern is reassuring, continued labor induction beyond 12 hours in the latent phase is reasonable and allows some women to achieve vaginal delivery without imperiling themselves or their fetus.

ACTIVE PHASE DISORDERS

Practically speaking, a parturient usually enters the active phase of labor when cervical dilation reaches 4 cm. This phase of labor is characterized by contractions that increase in intensity, frequency, and duration accompanied by more rapid cervical change.

Abnormal labor definitions in the active phase were initially based on Friedman's original work from the 1950s. Hendricks and colleagues[13] published a paper in 1970 that challenged Friedman's conclusions about the course of normal human labor. They reported absence of the deceleration phase and noted similar rates of dilatation after 4 cm in nulliparas and multiparas. More recently, Zhang and colleagues[14] assessed labor in 1329 term nulliparas who entered labor spontaneously and delivered vaginally. They found that the cervix dilated more slowly in the active phase than reported by Friedman, taking twice as long on average to progress from 4 cm to 10 cm (5.5 versus 2.5 hours). Like Hendricks, Zhang and colleagues reported absence of the deceleration phase. Instead, they reported that as cervical dilation advanced, the rate of dilation actually increased (**Table 1**). In many of the patients who achieved vaginal delivery, the rate of change never exceeded 1 cm/h. Consistent with the historical evolution of labor management, 50% of women in the Zhang cohort received oxytocin versus only 9% in Friedman's group.[14]

Based on the work of Friedman, protracted active phase traditionally has been defined as cervical dilatation less than 1.2 cm/h for nulliparas and less than 1.5 cm/h for multiparas.[7] In 1994, the World Health Organization proposed a labor management schema in which protraction is defined as cervical dilation less than 1 cm/h for 4 hours.[15] Arrested active phase traditionally has been defined as the absence of cervical change for 2 hours or more in the presence of adequate uterine contractility. In 1989, the American College of Obstetricians and Gynecologists suggested that arrest

Table 1 Expected time to make 1 centimeter of labor progress based on starting cervical dilation			
Cervical Dilation (cm)		—	
From	To	Median Time (h)	5th, 95th Percentiles (h)
2	3	3.2	0.6, 15.0
3	4	2.7	0.6, 10.1
4	5	1.7	0.4, 6.6
5	6	0.8	0.2, 3.1
6	7	0.6	0.2, 2.2
7	8	0.5	0.1, 1.5
8	9	0.4	0.1, 1.3
9	10	0.4	0.1, 1.4

Data from Zhang Troendle J, Yancey M. Reassessing the labor curve in nulliparous women. Am J Obstet Gynecol 2002;187(4):824–8.

cannot be diagnosed until both of the following criteria are met: (1) the latent phase has been completed with the cervix dilated 4 cm or more and (2) a uterine contraction pattern of 200 Montevideo units or more has been present for 2 hours without cervical change.[16] The following studies challenge the 2-hour timeframe and illustrate that vaginal delivery can be achieved despite slower labor progress without increasing adverse maternal or neonatal outcomes. These contemporary data should prompt reconsideration of the current recommendation.

In 1987, Arulkumarin and colleagues[17] prospectively analyzed the progress of labor in 220 nulliparous and 99 multiparous women who presented in spontaneous labor. This group sought to evaluate the benefit (measured in terms of mode of delivery and neonatal condition) in prolonging the oxytocin augmentation period for another 4 hours in patients with unsatisfactory progress after an initial period of 4 hours' augmentation. Women were recruited to the study once they reached the active phase of labor (defined as 3 cm dilation). Four hours later, the cervix was re-evaluated. If the progress of labor was less than expected (< 1 cm/h for 4 hours), dysfunctional labor was diagnosed and oxytocin augmentation was started. Four hours after the initiation of oxytocin, the patient was re-examined. If labor progress resumed at 1 cm of dilation or more per hour, the dysfunctional labor was deemed corrected. If not, the patient was considered to have abnormal progress and oxytocin was continued for an additional 4 hours. In women with adequate progress after oxytocin augmentation, 84.6% delivered vaginally, and no infants had Apgar scores less than 6 at 5 minutes. In a subgroup that had continued abnormal progress after the initial 4 hours of augmentation and received at least 4 additional hours of oxytocin, 25% delivered vaginally, and no infants had Apgar scores less than 6 at 5 minutes. In nulliparas, a period of 8 hours of augmentation resulted in an 18.2% cesarean delivery rate and no cases of birth injury or birth asphyxia, whereas if the period of augmentation were limited to 4 hours, the cesarean delivery rate would have nearly doubled (35.5%).[17]

In 1999, Rouse and colleagues[18] saw the potential for reducing the number of cesarean deliveries by adopting a more stringent definition of dystocia (specifically, active phase labor arrest). To that end, they assessed a labor management protocol that mandated at least 4 hours of postarrest oxytocin augmentation with adequate contractions ($\geq$ 200 Montevideo units) and 6 hours in the absence of adequate uterine contractions before cesarean delivery could be performed. The authors studied more than 500 women, and safe vaginal delivery was achieved in 92%. They demonstrated that extending the minimum period of oxytocin augmentation for active phase arrest from 2 hours to at least 4 hours was effective and safe and allowed most women studied to achieve vaginal delivery.[18] Although this study showed no significant increase in serious morbidty, it was of insufficient size to exclude an increased risk of some of the less frequent birth complications.

Subsequently, in 2001, the same group designed a study to provide contemporary, validated uterine activity and labor progress data from women receiving oxytocin for protracted or active phase arrest. By prospectively evaluating a cohort of 501 women, they were able to demonstrate that oxytocin-augmented labor proceeds at substantially slower rates than spontaneous labor and validated their previous work, which supported the contention that 2 hours of postactive phase arrest augmentation is insufficiently rigorous for the performance of cesarean delivery, despite at least 200 Montevideo units. In 286 nulliparous women undergoing pitocin augmentation, 235 delivered vaginally. In those women, the 10th percentile for cervical dilation per hour was 0.6 cm. Only 51 nulliparous women in that study required cesarean delivery, and they dilated significantly more slowly: 0.3 cm/h. Multiparous women who delivered vaginally dilated on average 1.8 cm/h, with the 10th percentile also at 0.6 cm/h.[19]

These data demonstrate that contemporary augmented labor that eventuates in vaginal delivery proceeds at substantially slower rates than spontaneous labor and is much slower than what Friedman traditionally defined. This finding suggests that traditional definitions should not apply to augmented or epidural-modified labor and that interventions based on traditional parameters will lead to unnecessary cesarean delivery. As illustrated in multiple contemporary studies, the definitions of abnormal labor may be too stringent for nulliparous women—especially when undergoing labor induction—and may contribute to unnecessary cesarean deliveries. Given these recent data, in the absence of other indications for expeditious delivery (eg, nonreassuring fetal heart rate), continued oxytocin augmentation in the face of active phase labor arrest is reasonable for at least 4 to 6 hours.

SECOND STAGE DISORDERS

The second stage of labor begins when the cervix becomes fully dilated and ends with delivery of the infant. The mean duration of the second stage is 54 minutes for nulliparas and 19 minutes for multiparas.[3] The upper limit of normal duration, or prolonged second stage, as traditionally defined is 3 hours (epidural) or 2 hours (no epidural) for nulliparas and 2 hours (epidural) or 1 hour (no epidural) without progressive descent of the presenting part.[20]

The concept that labor should be terminated if the duration of the second stage exceeds a specific amount of time depending on parity and presence of regional anesthesia has been ingrained in obstetric practice since the early 1800s. In 1952, Hellman and Prystowsky[21] reported an increase in neonatal death, postpartum hemorrhage, and puerperal infection when the second stage of labor exceeded 2 hours. More recent studies from the era of continuous electronic fetal monitoring have suggested that adverse neonatal outcomes are not influenced by the length of the second stage,[22,23] but the success rate of vaginal delivery decreases substantially after 3 hours,[24] and rates of maternal morbidities, including chorioamnionitis, perineal trauma, operative vaginal delivery, and postpartum hemorrhage, rise after 2 hours. Numerous factors affect the length of the second stage. For example, the use of regional anesthesia can increase the length of the second stage by 30 minutes.[25] Parity, maternal size, birth weight, occiput posterior position, and fetal station at complete dilation have been shown to affect the length of the second stage.[26] Several authors have specifically examined the relationship between length of second stage and adverse maternal and neonatal outcomes.

In 1976, Cohen[27] analyzed obstetric data from 4400 women and found no significant increase in the frequency of perinatal mortality, neonatal mortality, or low 5-minute Apgar scores with progressive lengthening of the second stage, regardless of delivery type, presence of maternal disease, or abnormal labor. An increase in the incidence of low 1-minute Apgar scores was observed only in cases in which fetal heart rate monitoring was not used. Postpartum hemorrhage increased significantly after more than 3 hours and occurred more often in women whose prolonged second stages were terminated by cesarean delivery or midforceps. When stratified for delivery procedure, no such increases were seen in vaginal deliveries—even after more than 3 hours of second stage duration. Maternal febrile morbidity increased when the second stage was prolonged beyond 3 hours. When patients who delivered via cesarean were excluded from analysis, there was no difference in febrile morbidity among the various second stage duration groups. Cohen[27] concluded that there is no indication for electively terminating labor because an arbitrary period of time has elapsed in the second stage, as long as there is no evidence of significant fetal hypoxia (assuming descent is normal and there is no suggestion of fetopelvic disproportion).

In 1995, Menticoglou and colleagues[23] reported on the perinatal outcomes of 6041 labors that reached the second stage with a live fetus weighing 2500 g or more. This group retrospectively reviewed the perinatal morbidity and mortality as it related to duration of the second stage. The second stage lasted more than 3 hours in 11% of nulliparous women and more than 5 hours in 2.7%. There were no deaths among nonanomalous neonates, and there was no increase in the rate of neonatal seizures. The rates of low 5-minute Apgar scores tended to increase with increasing duration of the second stage; however, the rate of admission to the neonatal intensive care unit for low Apgar scores or low cord pH increased progressively up until 2 hours was reached and then went unchanged until 5 hours of second stage duration. Even if undelivered after 5 hours, only 1.2% of the infants were admitted to the neonatal intensive care unit. This group concluded that appropriately grown fetuses who are not compromised and enter the second stage in good condition seldom suffer from asphyxia if carefully monitored, even when the second stage is prolonged.[23]

In 2003, Myles and Santolaya[28] evaluated maternal and neonatal outcomes with a prolonged second stage of labor defined as longer than 120 minutes. More than 6000 women were prospectively analyzed. These women were grouped according to length of the second stage. Vaginal delivery rates were 98.7% when the second stage lasted less than 120 minutes, 84% when the second stage lasted longer than 120 minutes, 90.2% when the second stage lasted between 121 and 240 minutes, and 65.5% when the second stage lasted longer than 240 minutes. The women whose second stage lasted longer than 120 minutes had higher rates of perineal trauma, episiotomy usage, chorioamnionitis, postpartum hemorrhage, and operative vaginal delivery when compared with women whose second stage was less than 120 minutes. There were no significant differences in neonatal morbidities. Slightly more infants in the prolonged second stage group required admission to the neonatal intensive care unit, but this did not translate into prolonged hospital stay. The rate of shoulder dystocia was low at 1.3% for women whose second stage lasted between 121 and 240 minutes and 3.2% for women whose second stage duration was more than 240 minutes. The authors concluded that a prolonged second stage is associated with a high rate of vaginal delivery but an increased rate of maternal morbidity. There was no relationship between duration of the second stage and adverse neonatal outcomes.[28]

In 2004, Cheng and colleagues[29] retrospectively analyzed more than 15,000 nulliparous women who delivered vaginally. They observed no association between short-term neonatal morbidity and duration of the second stage, even when prolonged up to 6 hours. The rates of cesarean delivery, postpartum hemorrhage, third- and fourth-degree perineal lacerations, and operative vaginal delivery increased with increasing duration of the second stage. The increasing maternal morbidity was evident when the second stage progressed beyond 4 hours. What is most notable is that even when the second stage was prolonged longer than 4 hours, the cesarean delivery rate was only 33% (although the operative vaginal delivery rate was 50%).[29]

In 2007, Cheng and colleagues[30] examined perinatal outcomes associated with the second stage of labor in more than 5000 multiparous women. Duration of the second stage was stratified into hourly intervals. Most women (79.7%) delivered between 0 and 1 hour, and only 5% had second stages that lasted 3 hours or longer. Approximately 90% of women who had second stage duration between 0 and 2 hours achieved spontaneous vaginal delivery. In the subgroup of parous women who experienced a second stage of labor lasting longer than 2 hours, there was a higher risk of operative delivery, third- and fourth-degree perineal lacerations, and adverse neonatal outcomes. This same relationship was not observed in nulliparous women, which suggested that perhaps a long second stage in this small subgroup of multiparas may be a manifestation of true cephalopelvic disproportion or fetal malposition.[30]

A consensus for the optimal management of abnormal labor in the second stage is lacking. Ideally, management should maximize the achievement of vaginal delivery while minimizing adverse maternal and neonatal outcomes. The American College of Obstetricians and Gynecologists has advised that "the length of the second stage of labor is not in itself an absolute or even strong indication for operative termination of labor."[31] Based on the available data, in nulliparous women, the length of the second stage is not related to adverse neonatal outcomes. Adverse maternal outcomes are not evident until the second stage progresses beyond 3 hours.

SUMMARY

The complex interactions among the powers, the passenger, and the passage determine whether the fetus successfully negotiates the pelvis and delivers vaginally. When abnormalities of one or more of these processes occur, evaluation and treatment of their cause are necessary. Cesarean delivery is indicated at any stage in the labor process in the presence of nonreassuring fetal status or when conservative measures (eg, oxytocin administration) fail in the setting of abnormal labor. Traditionally held definitions of abnormal labor are less relevant to current obstetric practice, however. Several studies have re-evaluated the Friedman curve and the treatment recommendations based on his studies and have found no increase in adverse maternal or neonatal outcomes when additional time is allowed to elapse before a cesarean delivery is performed. The lack of consensus on definitions and optimal management strategies makes patient individualization necessary.

In reviewing the available, contemporary literature, definitions of various labor abnormalities that are sufficient to warrant cesarean delivery have been outlined (Table 2). In the absence of maternal or fetal indications for expedited delivery, cesarean delivery is not indicated for latent phase disorders. Cesarean delivery for failed induction seems acceptable but not mandatory if the active phase (defined as 4 cm of dilation, 90% effacement, or 5 cm regardless of effacement) has not been reached despite at least 12 hours of oxytocin after membrane rupture. In the active phase, cesarean delivery for labor arrest should not be performed unless oxytocin to alleviate the

Table 2			
Proposed guidelines for management of labor abnormalities[a]			
Abnormality	**Traditional Definition**	**Proposed Guidelines**	**Intervention[a]**
Protracted latent phase	>20 h nullipara >14 h multipara	Wide variation, no arbitrary cutoff	Expectant management, therapeutic rest
Failed induction	—	Active phase not reached despite amniotomy followed by 12 hours of oxytocin	Cesarean delivery versus continued induction
Protracted active phase	<1.2 cm/h nullipara <1.5 cm/h multipara	<0.6 cm/h nullipara <0.6 cm/h multipara	Amniotomy, placement of IUPC, oxytocin
Arrested active phase	No cervical change in 2 h with adequate contractions	No cervical change in 4 h despite adequate uterine activity using oxytocin or 6 h without adequate uterine activity using oxytocin	Cesarean delivery versus continued oxytocin augmentation
Protracted second stage	Descent <1 cm/h nullipara or <2 cm/h multipara	Lack of demonstrable progressive descent in 4 h	Oxytocin, maternal expulsive efforts
Arrested second stage	No descent after 2 h	No descent after 2 h	Operative vaginal delivery or cesarean delivery

[a] Assumes no abnormalities of the fetal heart rate or other contraindications for continued trial of labor or operative vaginal delivery.
   Data from references[32–39].

arrest has been administered for at least 4 hours. When to intervene for protracted labor is arguable, but slow rates of labor progress (eg, 0.6 cm/h) are consistent with safe vaginal delivery. Cesarean delivery in the second stage should be avoided for at least 4 hours if there is progressive fetal descent.

REFERENCES

1. Gabbe SG, Niebyl JR, Simpson JL. Obstetrics: normal and problem prengancies. 5th edition. New York: Churchill Livingstone; 2007.
2. Zhu BP, Grigorescu V, Le T, et al. Labor dystocia and its association with interpregnancy interval. Am J Obstet Gynecol 2006;195(1):121–8.
3. American College of Obstetricians and Gynecologists. Dystocia and augmentation of labor. ACOG practice bulletin number 49. Obstet Gynecol 2003;102:1445–54.
4. Cunningham FG, Gant NF, Leveno KJ, et al. Williams obstetrics. 22nd edition. New York: McGraw-Hill; 2005.
5. Friedman E. The graphic analysis of labor. Am J Obstet Gynecol 1954;68:1568–75.

6. Blackwell SC, Refuerzo J, Chadha R, et al. Duration of labor induction in nulliparous women at term: how long is long enough? Am J Perinatol 2008;25: 205–9.
7. Sokol R, Stojkow BS, Chik L, et al. Normal and abnormal labor progress: I. A quantitative assessment and survey of the literature. J Reprod Med 1977;18:47–53.
8. Rinehart B, Terrone D, Hudson C, et al. Lack of utility of standard labor curves in the prediction of progression during labor induction. Am J Obstet Gynecol 2000; 182:1520–6.
9. Martin J, Hamilton B, Sutton P, et al. Births: final data for 2004. National Vital Statistics Reports 2006;55(1):1–102.
10. Lin M, Rouse D. What is a failed labor induction? Clin Obstet Gynecol 2006;49(3): 585–93.
11. Rouse DJ, Owen J, Hauth JC. Criteria for failed labor induction: prospective evaluation of a standardized protocol. Obstet Gynecol 2000;96(5 Pt 1):671–7.
12. Simon CE, Grobman WA. When has an induction failed? Obstet Gynecol 2005; 105(4):705–9.
13. Hendricks CH, Brenner WF, Kraus G. Normal cervical dilation pattern in late pregnancy and labor. Am J Obstet Gynecol 1970;106:1065–80.
14. Zhang J, Troendle J, Yancey M. Reassessing the labor curve in nulliparous women. Am J Obstet Gynecol 2002;187(4):824–8.
15. Lennox C, Kwast B. Preventing prolonged labor I. World Health Organization; 1994.
16. American College of Obstetricians and Gynecologists. Dystocia. ACOG technical bulletin number 137. Washington, DC: American College of Obstetricians and Gynecologists; 1989.
17. Arulkumaran S, Koh CH, Ingemarsson I, et al. Augmentation of labor: mode of delivery related to cervicometric progress. Aust N Z J Obstet Gynaecol 1987;27: 304–8.
18. Rouse DJ, Owen J, Hauth J. Active-phase labor arrest: oxytocin augmentation for at least 4 hours. Obstet Gynecol 1999;93(3):323–7.
19. Rouse DJ, Owen J, Savage K, et al. Active phase labor arrest: revisiting the 2-hour minimum. Obstet Gynecol 2001;98(4):550–4.
20. American College of Obstetricians and Gynecologists. Operative vaginal delivery. ACOG practice bulletin number 17. Obstet Gynecol 2000.
21. Hellman LM, Prystowsky H. The duration of the second stage of labor. Am J Obstet Gynecol 1952;63:1223–33.
22. Moon JM, Smith CV, Rayburn WE. Perinatal outcome after a prolonged second stage of labor. J Reprod Med 1990;35:229–31.
23. Menticoglou SM, Manning F, Harman C, et al. Perinatal outcome in relation to second-stage duration. Am J Obstet Gynecol 1995;173:906–12.
24. Friedman EA, Sachtleben MR. Dysfunctional labor. III. Secondary arrest of dilatation in the nullipara. Obstet Gynecol 1962;19:576–91.
25. Zhang J, Yancey MK, Klebanoff MA, et al. Does epidural analgesia prolong labor and increase risk of cesarean delivery? A natural experiment. Am J Obstet Gynecol 2001;185:128–34.
26. Piper JM, Bolling DR, Newton ER. The second stage of labor: factors influencing duration. Am J Obstet Gynecol 1991;165:976–9.
27. Cohen W. Influence of the duration of second stage labor on perinatal outcome and puerperal morbidity. Obstet Gynecol 1976;49(3):266–9.
28. Myles TD, Santolaya J. Maternal and neonatal outcomes in patients with a prolonged second stage of labor. Obstet Gynecol 2003;102(1):52–8.

29. Cheng YW, Hopkins LM, Caughey AB. How long is too long: does a prolonged second stage of labor in nulliparous women affect maternal and neonatal outcomes? Am J Obstet Gynecol 2004;191:933–8.

30. Cheng YW, Hopkins LM, Laros RK, et al. Duration of second stage labor in multiparous women: maternal and neonatal outcomes. Am J Obstet Gynecol 2007; 196:585.e1–6.

31. Caldeyro-Barcia R, Alvarez H, Reynolds S. A better understanding of uterine contractility through simultaneous recording with an internal and seven channel external method. Surg Gynecol Obstet 1950;91:641–50.

32. Sharma SK, Sidawi JE, Ramin SM, et al. Cesarean delivery: a randomized trial of epidural versus patient-controlled meperidine analgesia during labor. Anesthesiology 1997;87:472–6.

33. Thorp JA, Parisi VM, Boylan PC, et al. The effect of continuous epidural analgesia on cesarean section for dystocia in nulliparous women. Am J Obstet Gynecol 1989;161:670–5.

34. Alexander JM, Leveno KJ, Rouse DJ, et al. Comparison of maternal and infant outcomes from primary cesarean delivery during the second compared with first stage of labor. Obstet Gynecol 2007;109:917–21.

35. Satin AJ, Maberry MC, Leveno KJ, et al. Chorioamnionitis: a harbinger of dystocia. Obstet Gynecol 1992;79(6):913–5.

36. Friedman EA, Sachtleben MR. Dysfunctional labor V. Therapeutic trial of oxytocin in secondary arrest. Obstet Gynecol 1963;21:13–21.

37. Lin M, Reid K, Treaster M, et al. Transcervical Foley catheter with and without extraamniotic saline infusion for labor induction: a randomized controlled trial. Obstet Gynecol 2007;110(3):558–65.

38. Friedman E. Labor in multiparas. Obstet Gynecol 1956;9:691–703.

39. Ramin SM, Gambling DR, Lucas MJ, et al. Randomized trial of epidural versus intravenous analgesia during labor. Obstet Gynecol 1995;86:783–9.

Vaginal Birth After Cesarean Delivery

Mark B. Landon, MD

KEYWORDS

• VBAC • Trial of labor • Repeat cesarean

More than 25 year ago, It was recognized that a primary emphasis should be placed on reducing cesarean deliveries for dystocia and repeat operations because these two indications were the most significant causes of an escalating national rate of cesarean deliveries.[1] A panel of experts convened by a 1981 National Institute of Child Health and Human Development (NICHD)-sponsored conference also recognized the importance of decreasing elective repeat operations as a means of curtailing the rising overall cesarean rate.[2] A modest decline in cesarean delivery then followed between 1988 and 1996, which was largely due to an increased trial of labor (TOL) rate in women with prior cesareans. However, by 2004, only 9.2% of women with prior cesarean underwent a TOL in the United States.[3] Remarkably, it has been estimated that nearly two thirds of women with a prior cesarean are actually candidates for a TOL.[4] Thus, most repeat operations can be considered elective and are clearly influenced by physician practice style.[5] TOL rates are consistently lower in the United States when compared with European nations, suggesting significant underutilization of TOL in this country.[6] Because 8% to 10% of the obstetric population has experienced prior cesarean delivery, more widespread use of TOL could decrease the overall cesarean delivery rate by approximately 5%.[7]

The evolution in management of the woman with prior cesarean delivery is apparent through a review of several American College of Obstetricians and Gynecologists (ACOG) documents and key studies over the last 15 years. In 1988, ACOG published "Guidelines for vaginal delivery after a previous cesarean birth," endorsing vaginal birth after cesarean delivery (VBAC)-TOL as it became clear that this procedure was safe and did not appear to be associated with appreciable excess perinatal morbidity, compared with elective cesarean delivery. They recommended that each hospital develop its own protocol for the management of VBAC-TOL patients and that a woman with one prior low transverse cesarean delivery should be counseled and encouraged to attempt labor in the absence of a contraindication such as a prior classic incision. This recommendation was supported by several large case series attesting to the

Department of Obstetrics and Gynecology, Division of Maternal-Fetal Medicine, The Ohio State University College of Medicine, Means Hall – Room 509, 395 W. 12th Avenue, Columbus, OH 43210-1228, USA
E-mail address: landon.1@osu.edu

Clin Perinatol 35 (2008) 491–504
doi:10.1016/j.clp.2008.07.004
0095-5108/08/$ – see front matter © 2008 Elsevier Inc. All rights reserved.

safety and effectiveness of TOL.[8-12] Driven by this encouraging information, VBAC rates reached a peak of 28.3% by 1996. Third-party payors and managed care organizations embraced these data and began to encourage TOLs for women with prior cesarean delivery by tracking provider and institutional VBAC rates as a measure of quality. Physicians, feeling pressure to lower cesarean delivery rates, began to offer TOL liberally and in doing so may have included less than optimal candidates.

With greater use of VBAC-TOLs, reports began to surface suggesting a potentially greater than previously appreciated risk for uterine rupture and its maternal and fetal consequences.[13-17] Descriptions of uterine rupture with maternal hemorrhage, hysterectomy, and adverse perinatal outcomes, including death and brain injury, then set the stage for the precipitous decline in VBAC witnessed during the last decade.[18-21]

Eventually, ACOG acknowledged the apparent statistically small but significant risks for uterine rupture with poor outcomes for women and their infants during TOLs.[22] It was also recognized that such adverse events during a TOL might precipitate malpractice litigation. A more conservative approach to TOL has thus been adopted by even ardent supporters of VBAC. Nonetheless, ACOG, in its 2004 Bulletin, states clearly that most women with one previous cesarean delivery with a low transverse incision are candidates for VBAC and should be counseled about VBAC and offered a TOL.[23]

SELECTING CANDIDATES FOR A TRIAL OF LABOR

Women who have had low transverse uterine incision with prior cesarean delivery and have no contraindications to vaginal birth can be considered candidates for TOL. The following are criteria suggested by ACOG[23] for identifying candidates:

One previous low transverse cesarean delivery
Clinically adequate pelvis
No other uterine scars or previous rupture
Physicians immediately available throughout active labor capable of monitoring labor and performing an emergency cesarean delivery

The recommendation for having a physician "immediately available" and the implication that anesthesia service for emergency cesarean be present around the clock have significantly limited access to VBAC-TOL in rural hospitals.

Several retrospective studies would indicate that it may be reasonable to offer a TOL to women in several other clinical situations. These would include two previous low transverse cesarean deliveries, gestation beyond 40 weeks, previous low vertical incision, unknown uterine scar type, and twin gestation.[23]

A TOL is contraindicated in women at high risk for uterine rupture and should not be attempted in following circumstances:

Previous classic or T-shaped incision or extensive transfundal uterine surgery
Previous uterine rupture
Medical or obstetric complications that preclude vaginal delivery
Inability to perform emergency cesarean delivery because of unavailable surgeon or anesthesia, or insufficient staff or faculty.

SUCCESS RATES FOR TRIAL OF LABOR

The overall success rate for VBAC appears to be in the 70% to 80% range, according to published reports.[24-26] However, in published series with the highest TOL rates, only 60% of cases were successful.[27] More recently, selective criteria resulting in

TOL rates in the 30% range have been associated with a higher number of vaginal births (70%–75%).[28,29] Several predictors of successful TOL have been well described (**Table 1**). The prior indication for the cesarean delivery clearly impacts the likelihood of successful VBAC. A history of prior vaginal birth or a nonrecurring condition such as breech or fetal distress is associated with the highest success rates for VBAC (see **Table 1**).[10] Recently, Grobman and colleagues[30] have developed a nomogram for predicting VBAC. The prediction model is based on a multivariable logistic regression, including the variables of maternal age, body mass index, ethnicity, prior vaginal delivery, the occurrence of a VBAC, and a potentially recurrent indication for the cesarean delivery. After analyzing the model with cross validation techniques, it was found to be accurate and discriminating. Several factors have been studied that influence success and these are summarized in the following sections.

Maternal Demographics

Race, age, body mass index, and insurance status have all been demonstrated to impact the success of TOL.[28] In a multicenter study of 14,529 term pregnancies undergoing TOL, Caucasian women had an overall 78% success rate compared with 70% in non-Caucasian women.[28] Obese women are more likely to fail a TOL, as are women older than age 40.[28] Women who have a BMI greater than 40 have a 60.7% success rate, compared with a 77.7% success rate for those who have a BMI of 25.0 to 29.9.[31] Conflicting data exist with regard to payor status (uninsured versus private patients).

Prior Indication for Cesarean Delivery

Success rates for women whose first cesarean delivery was performed for a nonrecurring indication (breech, nonreassuring fetal well-being) are similar to vaginal delivery rates among nulliparous women.[32] Prior cesarean for breech presentation is associated with the highest reported success rate of 89%.[28,32] In contrast, prior operative delivery for cephalopelvic disproportion/failure to progress is associated with success rates ranging from 50% to 67%.[33,34] Hoskins and Gomez[35] have reported that if dystocia was diagnosed between 5 and 9 cm in a prior labor, 67% to 73% of VBAC attempts are successful, compared with only 13% if prior cesarean delivery was performed during the second stage of labor.

Prior Vaginal Delivery and Prior Vaginal Birth After Cesarean Delivery

Prior vaginal delivery, including prior successful VBAC, is apparently the strongest predictor of a successful TOL.[28] In one series, a prior vaginal delivery was associated with an 87% success rate, compared with 61% success in women without prior vaginal delivery.[28] Caughey and colleagues[36] reported patients with a prior VBAC had a 93% success rate, compared with 85% for women with a vaginal delivery prior to their cesarean birth, who were without prior VBAC. Mercer and colleagues[37] have noted that women with one prior successful TOL achieved an 87.6% success rate, compared with a 90.9% success rate for those with two prior successful attempts.

Birth Weight

Large-for-gestational-age or fetal macrosomia is associated with a lower likelihood of VBAC success.[29] Birth weight greater than 4000 g, in particular, is associated with a significantly higher risk for failed TOL.[28] Nonetheless, Flamm and Goings[38] reported that 60% to 70% of women who attempt VBAC with a macrosomic fetus are successful. Birth weight difference between first pregnancy (delivered by cesarean) and second pregnancy with attempted VBAC clearly influences successful rates. Peaceman

Table 1 Success rates for trial of labor	VBAC Success (%)
Prior indication	
CPD/FTP	63.5
NRFWB	72.6
Malpresentation	83.8
Prior vaginal delivery	
Yes	86.6
No	60.9
Labor type	
Induction	67.4
Augmented	73.9
Spontaneous	80.6

Abbreviations: CPD, cephalopelvic disproportion; FTP, failure to progress; NRFWB, nonreassuring fetal well-being.

Data from Landon MB, Leindecker S, Spong CY, et al. Factors affecting the success of trial of labor following prior cesarean delivery. Am J Obstet Gynecol 2005;193:1016–23.

and colleagues[39] reported a 34% success rate when the second pregnancy birth weight exceeded the first by 500 g and the prior indication was dystocia, compared with a 64% success rate with other prior indications.

Labor Status and Cervical Examinations

Labor status and cervical examination on admission influence VBAC success. An 86% VBAC success rate has been reported in women presenting with cervical dilation greater than or equal to 4 cm.[40] Conversely, the success rate drops to 67% if the cervical examination is less than 4 cm upon admission.

Women who undergo induction of labor are at higher risk for a failed TOL/repeat cesarean delivery compared with those who enter spontaneous labor.[28] Landon and colleagues[28] reported a 67.4% successful VBAC rate in women undergoing induction versus 80.6% in those entering spontaneous labor. Remarkably, Grinstead and Grobman reported a surprisingly high success rate (78%) in 429 women undergoing induction with prior cesarean delivery.[41] These authors noted several factors in addition to past obstetric history, including indication for induction and need for cervical ripening as determinants of VBAC success.[40] Grobman and colleagues[42] from the NICHD Maternal-Fetal Medicine Units (MFMU) Network have recently reported a VBAC success rate of 83% in 1298 women with a prior cesarean and prior vaginal delivery undergoing induction of labor.

Previous Incision Type

Previous incision type may be unknown in certain patients. It appears that women with unknown scar have VBAC success rates similar to those of women with documented prior low transverse incisions.[28] Similarly, women with previous low vertical incisions do not appear to have lower VBAC success rates.[43]

Multiple Prior Cesarean Deliveries

Women with more than one prior cesarean have been demonstrated to consistently have a lower likelihood of achieving VBAC.[44–46] Caughey and colleagues[44] reported a 75% success rate for women with one prior cesarean compared with 62% in women with two prior operations. In contrast, Macones' large multicenter study of 13,617 women undergoing a TOL revealed a 75.5% success rate for women with two prior cesareans, which was not statistically different from the 75% success rate in women with one prior operation (**Table 2**).[47]

RISKS FOR VAGINAL BIRTH AFTER CESAREAN DELIVERY–TRIAL OF LABOR
Uterine Rupture

The principal risk associated with VBAC-TOL is uterine rupture. This complication is directly attributable to attempted VBAC; symptomatic rupture is a rare observation at the time of elective repeat operations.[48,49] It is important to distinguish between uterine rupture and uterine scar dehiscence. This difference is clinically relevant because dehiscence most often represents an occult scar separation with intact serosa observed at laparotomy in women with a prior cesarean delivery. In cases of dehiscence, the potential for hemorrhage with fetal and maternal sequelae is absent. In contrast, uterine rupture is a through and through disruption of all uterine layers with consequences for potential hemorrhage, cord compression, abruption, fetal compromise, and significant maternal morbidity. The VBAC literature unfortunately varies with respect to terminology, definitions, and ascertainment for uterine rupture.[50] A review of 10 observational studies providing the best evidence on the occurrence of symptomatic rupture with TOL revealed rupture rates ranging from 0/1000 in a small study to 7.8/1000 in the largest study, with a pooled rate of 3.8 per 1000 trials of labor.[50,51] The large multicenter prospective observational MFMU Network study reported a 0.69% incidence, with 124 symptomatic ruptures occurring in 17,898 women undergoing TOL.[52]

The rate of uterine rupture depends on the type and location of the previous uterine incision (**Table 3**). Uterine rupture rates are highest with previous classic or T-shaped incisions, with a reported range of between 4% and 9%.[53] The risk for rupture with a previous low vertical incision has been difficult to determine. Distinguishing this incision type from classic incision can be arbitrary and the use of the low vertical incision is uncommon. Two reports suggest a rate of rupture of between 0.8% and 1.1% for prior low vertical scar.[53,54]

Women with unknown scar type may not be at increased risk for uterine rupture, which may simply represent the fact that most cases represent undocumented prior low transverse incisions. Among 3206 women with unknown scar in the MFMU Network cesarean registry, uterine rupture occurred in 0.5% of the TOLs.[52]

The most serious sequelae of uterine rupture include perinatal death, fetal hypoxic brain injury, and hysterectomy. Guise and colleagues[51] calculated a rate of 0.14 additional perinatal deaths per 1000 TOLs related to uterine rupture. This figure is remarkably similar to that in the NICHD MFMU Network study, in which two neonatal deaths occurred among 124 ruptures, for an overall rate of rupture-related perinatal death of 0.11 per 1000 trials of labor.[52] Chauhan and colleagues,[55] in reviewing 880 maternal

Table 2		
Success rates for trial of labor with two prior cesarean deliveries		
Author	**n**	**Success Rate (%)**
Miller[45]	2936	75.3
Caughey[44]	134	62.0
Macones[47]	1082	74.6
Landon[46]	876	67.0

Table 3	
Risk for uterine rupture with trial of labor	
Prior IncisionType	**Rupture Rate (%)**
Low transverse	0.5–1.0
Low vertical	0.8–1.1
Classic or T	4–9.0

uterine ruptures during a 20-year period, calculated 40 perinatal deaths in 91,039 TOLs, for a rate of 0.4 per 1000.

In most studies, perinatal hypoxic brain injury related to uterine rupture has been either underreported or poorly defined. Landon and colleagues[52] found a significant increase in the rate of hypoxic-ischemic encephalopathy (HIE) related to uterine rupture among the offspring of women who underwent a TOL at term, as compared with the children of women who underwent elective repeat cesarean delivery (0.46 per 1000 TOLs versus no cases, respectively). In 114 cases of uterine rupture at term, seven infants (6.2%) sustained HIE and two of these infants died in the neonatal period.

Maternal hysterectomy may be a complication of uterine rupture, particularly if the defect is unrepairable or is associated with uncontrollable hemorrhage. In five studies reporting on hysterectomies related to rupture, seven cases occurred in 60 symptomatic ruptures (13%; range 4%–27%), indicating that 3.4 per 10,000 women electing TOL sustain a rupture that necessitates hysterectomy.[50] The NICHD MFMU Network study included 5/124 (4%) rupture cases requiring hysterectomy in which the uterus could not be repaired.[52]

RISK FACTORS FOR UTERINE RUPTURE

Rates of uterine rupture vary significantly depending on various associated risk factors. In addition to uterine scar type, obstetric history characteristics, including number of prior cesareans, prior vaginal delivery, interdelivery interval, and uterine closure technique, have all been reported to affect the risk for uterine rupture. Similarly, factors related to labor management, including induction and the use of oxytocin augmentation, have all been studied. In contrast to predicting whether a TOL would be successful, Grobman and colleagues[56] could not develop a useful prediction model for uterine rupture that would be either accurate or discriminating.

Number of Prior Cesarean Deliveries

Miller and colleagues[45] reported uterine rupture in 1.7% of women with two or more previous cesarean deliveries, compared with a frequency of 0.6% in those with one prior operation (odds ratio 3.06; 95% confidence interval 1.95–4.79). The risk for uterine rupture was not increased further for women with three prior cesareans. Caughey and colleagues[44] conducted a smaller study of 134 women with two prior cesareans and controlled for labor characteristics and obstetric history. These investigators reported a rate of uterine rupture of 3.7% among these 134 women, compared with 0.8% in the 3757 women with one pervious scar (odds ratio 4.5; 95% confidence interval 1.18–11.5). This information likely led to the ACOG recommendation that TOL for women with two prior cesarean deliveries be limited to those with a history of prior vaginal delivery.[23] Recently, Macones and colleagues[47] reported a uterine rupture rate of 20/1082 (1.8%) in women with two prior cesareans, compared with 113/12,535 (0.9%) in women with one prior operation (adjusted odds ratio 2.3; 95% confidence interval 1.37–3.85). In contrast, an analysis from the MFMU Network cesarean registry found no significant difference in rupture rates in women with one prior cesarean (115/16,916 [0.7%]) versus those with multiple prior cesareans (9/982 [0.9%]).[47] Thus, it appears that if having multiple prior cesarean sections is associated with an increased risk for uterine rupture, the magnitude of any additional risk is fairly small (see **Table 3**).

Prior Vaginal Delivery

Prior vaginal delivery is protective against uterine rupture following TOL. Zelop and colleagues[57] noted the rate of uterine rupture among women with prior vaginal birth to be 0.2% (2/1021), compared with 1.1% (30/2762) among women with no prior vaginal deliveries. A similar protective effect of prior vaginal birth has been reported in two large multicenter studies.[47,58] Currently, no information exists as to whether a history of successful VBAC is also protective against uterine rupture.

Uterine Closure Technique

A single-layer uterine closure technique is commonly used because it is associated with a shorter operating time with similar short-term complications compared to the traditional two-layer technique. A retrospective study of 292 women undergoing TOL found similar rates of uterine rupture for women with one- and two-layer closures.[59] Chapman and colleagues[60] conducted a randomized trial that compared the incidence of uterine rupture among 145 women who received either one- or two-layer closure at their primary cesarean delivery. No cases of uterine rupture were found in either group; however, the study is of insufficient size to detect a potential difference. A large observational cohort study identified an approximate fourfold increased rate of rupture following single-closure technique when compared with previous double-layer closure.[61] These investigators conducted detailed review of operative reports in which the rate of rupture was 15/1489 (3.1%) with single-layer closure versus 8/1491 (0.5%) with previous double-layer closure. A large randomized study will be necessary to resolve whether single-layer closure increases the risk for subsequent uterine rupture.

Interpregnancy Interval

Short interpregnancy intervals have been studied as a risk factor for uterine rupture during TOLs.[62-64] Shipp and colleagues[62] reported an incidence of rupture of 2.3% (7/311) in women with an interdelivery interval of less than 18 months, compared with 1.1% (22/2098) with a longer interdelivery interval. In contrast, Huang and colleagues[63] found no increased risk for uterine rupture with an interdelivery interval of less than 18 months. Bujold and colleagues[64] have reported an interdelivery interval of less than 24 months to be independently associated with an almost threefold increased risk for uterine rupture. These investigators reported a rate of rupture of 2.8% in women with a short interval versus 0.9% in women for whom it was more than 2 years since the prior cesarean birth. Finally, Stamilio and colleagues[65] recently confirmed a similarly elevated rupture rate (2.7%) in women with less than 6 months between pregnancies, compared with 0.9% when the interpregnancy interval exceeded this time interval.

Labor Induction

Induction of labor appears be associated with an increased risk for uterine rupture.[52,58,66] In the prospective MFMU Network cohort analysis, Landon and co-workers[52] noted the risk for uterine rupture to be nearly threefold (elevated odds ratio 2.86; 95% confidence interval 1.75–4.67), with uterine rupture occurring after

48/4708 (1.0%) of induced TOLs versus 24/6685 (0.4%) of spontaneous labors. After controlling for various potential confounders, the risk for uterine rupture in women undergoing oxytocin labor induction has been reported to be increased 4.6-fold compared with spontaneous labor (rupture rate of 2.0% versus 0.7%).[57] Despite these analyses, it remains unclear whether induction causes uterine rupture or whether an associated risk factor such as cervical status is the ultimate cause. However, Grobman and colleagues[42] failed to detect a difference in rupture rates according to cervical status in women undergoing induction and TOL.

Conflicting data also exist as to whether various induction methods increase the risk for uterine rupture.[67] Lydon-Rochelle and associates'[66] study suggested an increased risk for uterine rupture with use of prostaglandins for labor induction. Uterine rupture was noted in 15/1960 (0.8%) of women induced without prostaglandin use, compared with 9/366 (2.5%) induced with prostaglandin use. Two recent large studies have failed to confirm these findings.[52,58] Macones and colleagues[58] did report an increased risk for rupture in women undergoing induction only if they received a combination of prostaglandins and oxytocin. The MFMU Network study had no cases of uterine rupture when prostaglandin alone was used for induction, including 52 cases of misoprostol use.[52] The safety of this medication, which is popular for cervical ripening and labor induction, has been challenged for women attempting VBAC. In a study from the Scottish Morbidity Record and the Stillborn and Infant Death Survey in Scotland, Smith and colleagues[68] reported a 0.87% risk for uterine rupture among 4475 women receiving prostaglandins, compared with 0.29% in 4429 cases not receiving this class of medication. Despite several studies that did not demonstrate an increased risk for rupture with prostaglandins and the fact that limited studies or meta-analyses have only detected a small statistically increased risk for rupture with misoprostol use, ACOG has issued a committee opinion discouraging the use of prostaglandins for cervical ripening or induction in women attempting VBAC-TOL until this issue is further clarified.[69]

Labor Augmentation

Excessive use of oxytocin may be associated with uterine rupture such that careful labor augmentation should be practiced in women attempting TOL. In a case-control study, Leung and colleagues[20] reported an odds ratio of 2.7 for uterine rupture in women receiving oxytocin augmentation. In contrast, a meta-analysis concluded that oxytocin does not increase the risk for uterine rupture.[10] Dysfunctional labor, including arrest disorders, actually increased the risk sevenfold and thus may actually be the primary factor responsible for rupture. In support of this concept, Zelop and colleagues[57] found that labor augmentation with oxytocin did not significantly increase the risk for rupture. In the MFMU Network study, the rate of uterine rupture with oxytocin augmentation was 52/6009 (0.9%), compared with 24/6685 (0.4%) without oxytocin use.[52] In summary, oxytocin augmentation may marginally increase the risk for uterine rupture in women undergoing TOL. It follows that judicious use of oxytocin should be used in this clinical setting.

MANAGEMENT OF VAGINAL BIRTH AFTER CESAREAN DELIVERY–TRIAL OF LABOR

Because uterine rupture may be catastrophic, it is recommended that TOL after prior cesarean delivery should only be attempted in institutions equipped to respond to emergencies, with physicians immediately available to provide emergent care.[23] Thus, an obstetrician and anesthesia personnel must be available to comply with this recommendation.

Recommendations for management of women undergoing a TOL after prior cesarean delivery are primarily based on expert opinion. Women attempting VBAC should be encouraged to contact their health care provider promptly when labor or ruptured membranes occur. Continuous electronic fetal heart rate monitoring is prudent, although the need for intrauterine pressure catheter monitoring is debatable. Studies that have examined fetal heart rate patterns prior to uterine rupture consistently report that nonreassuring signs, particularly significant variable decelerations or bradycardia, are the most common finding accompanying uterine rupture.[66,70] Despite the presence of adequate personnel to proceed with emergency cesarean delivery, prompt intervention does not always prevent fetal neurologic injury or death.[51,71] In one study, significant neonatal morbidity occurred when 18 minutes or longer elapsed between the onset of fetal heart rate deceleration and delivery.[20] If prolonged deceleration is preceded by variable or late decelerations, fetal injury may occur as early as 10 minutes from the onset of the terminal deceleration.

A TOL is not a contraindication to the use of epidural analgesia. Moreover, epidural use does not appear to affect success rates.[28] Epidural analgesia also does not mask the signs and symptoms of uterine rupture. Oxytocin augmentation is used as necessary, with the understanding that excess stimulation should be avoided. In a case-control study, Goetzl and colleagues[72] reported no association between uterine rupture and oxytocin dosing intervals, total dose used, and the mean duration of oxytocin administration.[72,73]

Vaginal delivery is conducted as in cases without a history of prior cesarean. Most individuals do not routinely explore the uterus in order to detect asymptomatic scar dehiscences because these generally heal well. However, excessive vaginal bleeding or maternal hypotension should be evaluated promptly, including assessment for possible uterine rupture. Of 124 cases of uterine rupture accompanying TOL in the MFMU cesarean registry, 14 (11%) were identified following vaginal delivery.[52]

COUNSELING FOR VAGINAL BIRTH AFTER CESAREAN DELIVERY–TRIAL OF LABOR

A pregnant woman with prior cesarean delivery is at risk for maternal and perinatal complications, whether undergoing TOL or choosing elective repeat operation. Complications of both procedures should be discussed and an attempt should be made to individualize the risk for uterine rupture and the likelihood of successful VBAC (**Table 4**). For example, a woman who might require induction of labor may be at a slightly increased risk for uterine rupture and is also less likely to achieve vaginal delivery. Future childbearing and the risks of multiple cesarean deliveries, including risks for placenta previa and accreta, should also be considered.

It is important to make every possible effort to obtain the operative records of a prior cesarean delivery to determine previous uterine incision type. This information is particularly relevant to cases of prior preterm breech delivery in which vertical uterine incision or a low transverse incision in an undeveloped lower uterine segment might preclude a TOL. Women with a prior preterm cesarean attempting TOL appear to have an increased rate of subsequent uterine rupture.[69,74] Sciscione and colleagues[73] have reported the risk for uterine rupture to be 1.18% with prior preterm cesarean delivery followed by term TOL. If previous uterine incision type is unknown, the implications of this missing information should also be discussed.

Following complete informed consent detailing the risks and benefits for the individual woman, the delivery plan should be formulated. Documentation of counseling is recommended and some practitioners prefer to use a specific VBAC consent form. Many women will elect repeat operation after thorough counseling. Regrettably,

Table 4
Comparison of maternal complications in trial of labor with elective repeat cesarean delivery

	Trial of Labor (n = 17,898)	Elective Repeat Cesarean Delivery (n = 15,801)	Odds Ratio (98% Confidence Interval)
Complication			
Uterine rupture	124 (0.70)	0	—
Hysterectomy	41 (0.20)	47 (0.30)	0.77 (0.51–1.17)
Thromboembolic disease	7 (0.04)	10 (0.10)	0.62 (0.24–1.62)
Transfusion	304 (1.70)	158 (1.00)	1.71 (1.41–2.08)
Endometritis	517 (2.90)	285 (1.80)	1.62 (1.40–1.87)
Maternal death	3 (0.02)	7 (0.04)	0.38 (1.10–1.46)
One or more of the above	978 (5.50)	563 (3.60)	1.56 (1.41–1.74)

Data from Landon MB, Hauth JC, Leveno KJ, et al for the National Institute of Child Health and Human Development Maternal-Fetal Medicine Units Network. Maternal and perinatal outcomes associated with a trial of labor after prior cesarean section. N Engl J Med 2004;351:2581–9.

bias is often introduced during counseling, as evidenced by a report detailing critical missing information being conveyed to women that differed depending on whether they elected TOL versus repeat operation.[75] However, VBAC-TOL should continue to remain an option for most women with prior cesarean delivery (**Box 1**). The magnitude of risks accompanying TOL must be disclosed. The attributable risk for a serious adverse perinatal outcome (perinatal death or HIE) at term appears to be approximately 1 in 2000 TOLs.[52] Combining an independent risk for hysterectomy attributable to uterine rupture at term with the risk for newborn HIE indicates the chance of one of these adverse events occurring to be approximately 1 in 1250 cases.[50]

Box 1
Risks associated with trial of labor versus elective repeat cesarean delivery

Risks associated with trial of labor

Uterine rupture and related morbidity

    Uterine rupture (0.5–1.0/100 TOL)

    Perinatal death and/or encephalopathy (0.5/1000 TOL)

    Hysterectomy (0.3/1000 TOL)

Increased maternal morbidity with failed TOL

    Transfusion

    Endometritis

    Length of stay

Potential risk for perinatal asphyxia with labor (cord prolapse, abruption)

Potential risk for antepartum stillbirth beyond 39 weeks gestation

Risks associated with elective repeat cesarean delivery

Increased maternal morbidity compared with successful TOL

Increased length of stay and recovery

Increased risks for abnormal placentation and hemorrhage with successive cesarean operations.

The decision to select a TOL may also increase the risk for perinatal death and HIE from labor-related events such as abruption and cord prolapse in the absence of uterine rupture. In the MFMU Network study, five cases of non–rupture-related HIE occurred in term infants in the TOL group, compared with none in the elective repeat cesarean population.[52] Additionally, for women awaiting spontaneous labor beyond 39 weeks, a small possibility exists of unexplained stillbirth, which would be theoretically avoidable with scheduled repeat operation.

REFERENCES

1. Bottoms SF, Rosen MG, Sokol RJ. The increase in the cesarean birth. N Engl J Med 1980;302:559.
2. Cesarean Childbirth: NICHD Consensus Development Conference. Washington, DC: DHHS Publication No. 81-2067, 1981.
3. Martin JA, Hamilton BE, Menachker F, et al. Preliminary births for. Health E-Stats. National Center for Health Statistics 2004. Available at: www.cdc.gov/nchs/products/pubs/pubd/hestats/prelimbirths/prelimbirths04.htm. Accessed June 1, 2008.
4. Flamm BL. Vaginal birth after cesarean section: controversies old and new. Clin Obstet Gynecol 1985;28:735.
5. Goldman G, Pineault R, Pitvin L, et al. Factors influencing the practice of vaginal birth after cesarean section. Am J Public Health 1993;83:1104.
6. Shiono PH, Fielden JR, McNellis D, et al. Recent trends in cesarean birth and trial of labor rates in the United States. JAMA 1987;257:494.
7. American College of Obstetricians and Gynecologists. Vaginal delivery after previous cesarean birth. Practice Patterns, No. 1. Washington, DC: ACOG; 1995.
8. Flamm BL, Newman LA, Thomas SJ, et al. Vaginal birth after cesarean delivery: results of a 5-year multicenter collaborative study. Obstet Gynecol 1990;76:750.
9. Flamm B, Goings J, Yunbao L, et al. Elective repeat cesarean section delivery versus trial of labor: a prospective multicenter study. Obstet Gynecol 1994;83:927.
10. Rosen MG, Dickinson JC, Westhoff CL. Vaginal birth after cesarean: a meta analysis of morbidity and mortality. Obstet Gynecol 1991;77:465.
11. Paul RH, Phelan JP, Yeh S. Trial of labor in the patient with a prior cesarean birth. Am J Obstet Gynecol 1985;151:297.
12. Martin JN Jr, Harris BA Jr, Huddleston JF, et al. Vaginal delivery following previous cesarean birth. Am J Obstet Gynecol 1983;146:255.
13. Beall M, Eglinton GS, Clark SL, et al. Vaginal delivery after cesarean section in women with unknown types of uterine scars. J Reprod Med 1984;29:31.
14. Pruett K, Kirshon B, Cotton D. Unknown uterine scar in trial of labor. Am J Obstet Gynecol 1988;159:807.
15. Scott J. Mandatory trial of labor after cesarean delivery: an alternative viewpoint. Obstet Gynecol 1991;77:811.
16. Pitkin RM. Once a cesarean? Obstet Gynecol 1991;77:939.
17. Sachs BP, Kobelin C, Castro MA, et al. The risks of lowering the cesarean-delivery rate. N Engl J Med 1990;340:54-7.
18. Farmer RM, Kirschbaum T, Potter D, et al. Uterine rupture during a trial of labor after previous cesarean section. Am J Obstet Gynecol 1991;165:996.
19. Boucher M, Tahilramaney MP, Eglinton GS, et al. Maternal morbidity as related to trial of labor after previous cesarean delivery: a quantitative analysis. J Reprod Med 1984;29:12.

20. Leung AS, Farmer RM, Leung EK, et al. Risk factors associated with uterine rupture during trial of labor after cesarean delivery: a case controlled study. Am J Obstet Gynecol 1993;168:1358.

21. Arulkumaran S, Chua S, Ratnam SS. Symptoms and signs with scar rupture— value of uterine activity measurements. Aust N Z J Obstet Gynaecol 1992;32:208.

22. Vaginal birth after previous cesarean delivery: clinical management guidelines for obstetricians-gynecologists. ACOG practice bulletin no. 5. Washington, DC: American College of Obstetricians and Gynecologists; 1999.

23. Vaginal birth after previous cesarean delivery: clinical management guidelines for obstetrician-gynecologists. ACOG Practice Bulletin No. 54. Washington, DC: American College of Obstetricians and Gynecologists; 2004.

24. Whiteside DC, Mahan SC, Cook JC. Factors associated with successful vaginal delivery after cesarean section. J Reprod Med 1983;28:785.

25. Silver RK, Gibbs RS. Prediction of vaginal delivery in patients with a previous cesarean section who require oxytocin. Am J Obstet Gynecol 1987;156:57.

26. Flamm BL. Vaginal birth after cesarean section. In: Flamm BL, Quilligan EJ, editors. Cesarean section: guidelines for appropriate utilization. New York: Springer-Verlog; 1995. p. 51–64.

27. Gregory KD, Korst LM, Cane P, et al. Vaginal birth after cesarean and uterine rupture rates in California. Obstet Gynecol 1999;93:985–9.

28. Landon MB, Leindecker S, Spong CY, For the National Institute of Child Health and Human Development Maternal-Fetal Medicine Units Network. The MFMU cesarean registry: factors affecting the success and trial of labor following prior cesarean delivery. Am J Obstet Gynecol 2005;193:1016–23.

29. Elkousky MA, Samuel M, Stevens E, et al. The effect of birthweight on vaginal birth after cesarean delivery success rates. Am J Obstet Gynecol 2003;188:824–30.

30. Grobman WA, Lai Y, Landon MB, et al. For the National Institute of Child Health and Human Development (NICHD) Maternal-Fetal Medicine Units Network (MFMU). Development of a nomogram for prediction of vaginal birth after cesarean delivery. Obstet Gynecol 2007;109(4):806–12.

31. Hibbard JU, Gilbert S, Landon MB, et al. For the National Institute of Child Health and Human Development (NICHD) Maternal-Fetal Medicine Units Network (MFMU). Trial of labor or repeat cesarean delivery in women with morbid obesity and previous cesarean delivery. Obstet Gynecol 2006;108(1):125–33.

32. Coughlan C, Kearney R, Turner MJ. What are the implications for the next delivery in primigravidae who have an elective cesarean section for breech presentation? BJOG 2002;109:624–6.

33. Ollendorff DA, Goldberg JM, Minoque JP, et al. Vaginal birth after cesarean section for arrest of labor: is success determined by maximum cervical dilatation during the prior labor? Am J Obstet Gynecol 1988;159:636.

34. Jongen VH, Halfwerk MG, Brouwer WK. Vaginal delivery after previous cesarean section for failure of second stage of labour. Br J Obstet Gynaecol 1998;195:1079.

35. Hoskins IA, Gomez JL. Correlation between maximum cervical dilation at cesarean delivery and subsequent vaginal birth after cesarean delivery. Obstet Gynecol 1997;89:591–3.

36. Caughey AB, Shipp TD, Repke JT, et al. Trial of labor after cesarean delivery: the effects of previous vaginal delivery. Am J Obstet Gynecol 1998;179:938–41.

37. Mercer BM, Gilbert S, Landon MB, et al. For the National Institute of Child Health and Human Development Maternal-Fetal Medicine Units Network. Labor

outcomes with increasing number of prior vaginal births after cesarean delivery. Obstet Gynecol 2008;111:285–91.

38. Flamm BL, Goings JR. Vaginal birth after cesarean section: is suspected fetal macrosomia a contraindication? Obstet Gynecol 1989;74:694.

39. Peaceman AM, Gersnoviez R, Landon MB, et al. For the NICHD Maternal-Fetal Medicine Units Network. The MFMU cesarean registry: impact of fetal size on trial of labor success for patients with prior cesarean for dystocia. Am J Obstet Gynecol 2006;195(4):1127–31.

40. Shipp TD, Zelop CM, Repke JT, et al. Labor after previous cesarean: influence of prior indication and parity. Obstet Gynecol 2000;95:913–6.

41. Grinstead J, Grobman WA. Induction of labor after one prior cesarean: predictors of vaginal delivery. Obstet Gynecol 2004;103(3):534–8.

42. Grobman WA, Gilbert S, Landon MB, et al. Outcomes of induction of labor after one prior cesarean. Obstet Gynecol 2007;109(2 PT1):262–9.

43. Rosen MG, Dickinson JC. Vaginal birth after cesarean: a meta analysis of indicators for success. Obstet Gynecol 1990;76:865.

44. Caughey AB, Shipp TD, Repke JT, et al. Rate of uterine rupture during a trial of labor in women with one or two prior cesarean deliveries. Am J Obstet Gynecol 1999;181:872–6.

45. Miller DA, Diaz FG, Paul RH. Vaginal birth after cesarean: a 10 year experience. Obstet Gynecol 1994;84:255–8.

46. Landon MB, Spong CY, Thom E, et al. For the NICHD Maternal-Fetal Medicine Units Network. The MFMU cesarean registry: risk of uterine rupture with a trial of labor in women with multiple and single prior cesarean delivery. Obstet Gynecol 2006;108:12–20.

47. Macones GA, Cahill A, Pare E, et al. Obstetric outcomes in women with two prior cesarean deliveries: is vaginal birth after cesarean delivery a viable option? Am J Obstet Gynecol 2005;192(4):1223–9.

48. Kieser KE, Baskett TF. A 10-year population-based study of uterine rupture. Obstet Gynecol 2002;100:749–53.

49. Mozurkewich EL, Hutton EK. Elective repeat cesarean delivery versus trial of labor: a meta-analysis of the literature from 1989 to 1999. Am J Obstet Gynecol 2000;183:1187–97.

50. Vaginal birth after cesarean (VBAC). Rockville (IN). Md.: Agency for Health Care Research and Quality; 2003. (AHRQ publication no. 03-E018.).

51. Guise JM, McDonagh MS, Osterweil P, et al. Systematic review of the incidence and consequences of uterine rupture in women with previous cesarean section. BMJ 2004;329:19–25.

52. Landon MB, Hauth JC, Leveno KJ, et al. For the National Institute of Child Health and Human Development Maternal-Fetal Medicine Units Network. Maternal and perinatal outcomes associated with a trial of labor after prior cesarean delivery. NEJM 2004;351:2581–9.

53. Naif RW 3rd, Ray MA, Chauhan SP, et al. Trial of labor after cesarean delivery with a lower-segment, vertical uterine incision: is it safe? Am J Obstet Gynecol 1995;172:1666–73.

54. Shipp TD, Zelop CM, Repke TJ, et al. Intrapartum uterine rupture and dehiscence in patients with prior lower uterine segment vertical and transverse incisions. Obstet Gynecol 1999;94:735–40.

55. Chauhan SP, Martin JN Jr, Henrichs CE, et al. Maternal and perinatal complications with uterine rupture in 142,075 patients who attempted vaginal birth after

cesarean delivery: a review of the literature. Am J Obstet Gynecol 2003;189: 408–17.

56. Grobman WA, Lai Y, Landon MB, et al. For the National Institute of Child Health and Human Development Maternal-Fetal Medicine Units Network. Prediction of uterine rupture associated with attempted vaginal birth after cesarean delivery. Am J Obstet Gynecol 2008;199(1):30.

57. Zelop CM, Shipp TD, Repke JT, et al. Uterine rupture during induced or augmented labor in gravid women with one prior cesarean delivery. Am J Obstet Gynecol 1999;181:882–6.

58. Macones G, Peipert J, Nelson D, et al. Maternal complications with vaginal birth after cesarean delivery: a multicenter study. Am J Obstet Gynecol 2005;193: 1656.

59. Tucker JM, Hauth JC, Hodgkins P, et al. Trial of labor after a one- or two-layer closure of a low transverse uterine incision. Obstet Gynecol 1993;168:545.

60. Chapman SJ, Owen J, Hauth JC. One- versus two-layer closure of a low transverse cesarean: the next pregnancy. Obstet Gynecol 1997;89:16–8.

61. Bujold E, Bujold C, Hamilton EF, et al. The impact of a single-layer or double-layer closure on uterine rupture. Am J Obstet Gynecol 2002;186:1326–30.

62. Shipp TD, Zelop CM, Repke JT, et al. Interdelivery interval and risk of symptomatic uterine rupture. Obstet Gynecol 2001;97:175–7.

63. Huang WH, Nakashima DK, Rummey PJ, et al. Interdelivery interval and the success of vaginal birth after cesarean delivery. Obstet Gynecol 2002;99:41–4.

64. Bujold E, Mehta SH, Bujold C, et al. Interdelivery interval and uterine rupture. Am J Obstet Gynecol 2002;187:199–202.

65. Stamilio D, DeFranco E, Pare E, et al. Short interpregnancy interval: risk of uterine rupture and complications of vaginal birth after cesarean delivery. Obstet Gynecol 2007;l10(5):1075–82.

66. Lydon-Rochelle M, Holt V, Easterling TR, et al. Risk of uterine rupture during labor among women with a prior cesarean delivery. N Engl J Med 2001;345:36–8.

67. Stone JL, Lockwood CJ, Berkowitz G, et al. Use of cervical prostaglandin E2 gel in patients with previous cesarean section. Am J Perinatol 1994;11:309–12.

68. Smith GC, Pell JP, Pasupathy D, et al. Factors predisposing to perinatal death related to uterine rupture during attempted vaginal birth after cesarean section: retrospective cohort study. BMJ 2004;14:329(7462):359–60.

69. ACOG Practice Bulletin. Induction of Labor. No 10, 1999.

70. Rodriguez M, Masaki D, Phelan J, et al. Uterine rupture: are intrauterine pressure catheters useful in the diagnosis? Am J Obstet Gynecol 1989;161:666.

71. Clark SL, Scott JR, Porter TF, et al. Is vaginal birth after cesarean less expensive than repeat cesarean delivery? Am J Obstet Gynecol 2000;182:599–602.

72. Goetzel L, Shipp TD, Cohen A, et al. Oxytocin dose and the risk of uterine rupture in trial of labor after cesarean. Obstet Gynecol 2001;97:381.

73. Sciscione A, Landon MB, Leveno KJ, et al. For the National Institute of Child Health and Human Development (NICHD) Maternal-Fetal Medicine Units Network (MFMU). Previous preterm cesarean delivery and risk of subsequent uterine rupture. Obstet Gynecol 2008;111:648–53.

74. Jones R, Nagashima A, Hartnett-Goodman M, et al. Rupture of low transverse cesarean scars during trial of labor. Obstet Gynecol 1991;77:815.

75. Renner RM, Eden KB, Osterweil P, et al. Informational factors influencing patient's childbirth preferences after prior cesarean. Am J Obstet Gynecol 2007;196(5): e14–6.

Cesarean Delivery on Maternal Request: the Impact on Mother and Newborn

Young Mi Lee, MD[a],*, Mary E. D'Alton, MD[b]

KEYWORDS

- Cesarean • Maternal request • Maternal morbidity
- Neonatal morbidity

Initially performed only for perimortem cases in ancient times, cesarean deliveries have now become one of the most commonly performed major abdominal surgeries. The most recent United States statistics estimate that in 2006, 1.3 million births, representing 31.1% of all deliveries, were via cesarean.[1] The rates for both primary and repeat cesareans have reached unprecedented highs and the number of vaginal birth after cesarean trials have dropped dramatically. Less clear is the degree of influence that cesarean deliveries on maternal request (CDMRs) have on this trend. Defined as a cesarean delivery on maternal request for a singleton pregnancy at term in the absence of medical or obstetric indications, CDMRs are estimated to make up 4% to 18% of all cesareans today.[2] The concept of CDMR not only reflects changing medical practice but also a shift in attitude by both health care practitioners and patients. Discussions about cesarean birth are never lacking in controversy or opinion and the debate has recently become increasingly heated, fueled by public awareness and speculation about the roles of medical, legal, and patient-choice issues as driving forces behind the high rates of cesarean births. In March 2006, the National Institute of Child Health and Human Development (NICHD), a branch of the National Institutes of Health (NIH), sponsored a state-of-the-science conference on CDMR to analyze and systematically review the current evidence, educate the public of the findings, and identify potential areas of future research.[2] The panel acknowledged that a large gap exists between current knowledge and clinical practice and expressed concern that this surgery is being chosen without rigorously evaluating the evidence. The

Mary E. D'Alton has worked as a consultant for Artemis Health, Inc., Menlo Park, California.

[a] Division of Maternal-Fetal Medicine, Department of Obstetrics and Gynecology, Weill Cornell Medical College, New York, NY, USA

[b] Department of Obstetrics and Gynecology, Columbia University Medical Center, New York, NY 10032, USA

* Corresponding author.

E-mail address: yml9002@med.cornell.edu (Y.M. Lee).

Clin Perinatol 35 (2008) 505–518
doi:10.1016/j.clp.2008.07.006
0095-5108/08/$ – see front matter © 2008 Elsevier Inc. All rights reserved.

data on CDMR, derived primarily from observational studies and extrapolated research, suggest that vaginal and cesarean deliveries are each associated with important risks and benefits. While the safest route of delivery may be an uncomplicated vaginal delivery, accurately predicting who will achieve this outcome is presently not possible. However, a CDMR performed before the onset of labor for a mother planning only one or two children may be reasonable after informed consent and counseling on the risks and benefits. Mothers contemplating a CDMR should be counseled that many of the potential risks of CDMR include complications in future pregnancies, with the understanding that, while future pregnancies may not be anticipated, more than half of all pregnancies are unplanned. The purpose of this article is to summarize the areas that should be reviewed in counseling patients about CDMR, focusing on the impact on mothers and newborns.

BENEFITS AND RISKS

An exhaustive query of injuries reputedly sustained during childbirth identifies such rare complications as fetal laryngeal rupture during vaginal delivery and maternal splenic rupture after cesarean.[3,4] Yet discussion of such risks are generally not included in routine counseling. Similarly, maternal request cesareans are associated with many potential benefits and risks, but any rational discussion on the topic should include only those risks and benefits that have a reasonable chance of occurring (**Box 1**). Potential medical risks that deserve mentioning include an increased risk of neonatal respiratory morbidity, potential surgical complications, and risks to future pregnancies, such as abnormal placentation and uterine rupture. Potential benefits include scheduling convenience, lower risk of hemorrhage, and decreased neonatal neurologic injury.

The primary advantage of cesarean by maternal request is avoiding an unplanned or emergent cesarean, which carries a higher risk for morbidity and psychologic trauma than a scheduled or planned cesarean.[2] On close examination, the paucity of evidence surrounding the majority of outcomes becomes clear and includes such common fears as pelvic floor injury, sexual dysfunction, thromboembolism, and mother-infant bonding.[2]

A variety of maternal and fetal outcomes were examined in the NIH conference, but an extensive literature search identified only five areas supported by moderate level evidence: maternal length of stay, hemorrhage, neonatal respiratory morbidity, subsequent placenta previa or accreta, and subsequent uterine rupture.[2,5] Although critical, the impact of CDMR on such outcomes as maternal and neonatal mortality are difficult to estimate because of their rarity. While a discussion of these risks and benefits should be thorough, providers are cautioned to avoid reciting a list of statistical probabilities, as many important and relevant factors may be difficult to examine or quantify.[6]

IMPACT ON MOTHER
Maternal Morbidity

Current literature suggests that term planned cesarean and planned vaginal deliveries have similar low absolute and relative rates of morbidity.[7] The largest and most recent randomized trial with proxy comparison groups is the Term Breech Trial. Hannah and colleagues[8] evaluated 2088 women from 121 centers in 26 countries with term (≥ 37 weeks), singleton, frank or complete breech fetuses weighing less than 4000 g, and no fetal anomalies. Of 1041 women scheduled for planned cesarean, 90.4% were delivered by cesarean, of which 50% presented in labor. Conversely, of 1042 women for

Box 1
Potential benefits and risks of CDMR

Maternal

Length of hospital stay[a]

Hemorrhage[a]

Pelvic floor injury

    Urinary incontinence

    Anorectal function

    Pelvic organ prolapse

    Sexual dysfunction

Future pregnancy

    Uterine rupture[a]

    Placenta previa and accreta[a]

    Fertility

    Stillbirth

Anesthesia complications

Infection

Surgical trauma

Hysterectomy

Thromboembolism

Postpartum pain

Depression

Maternal mortality

Fetal

Neonatal respiratory morbidity[a]

Breastfeeding

Neurologic injury

    Intracranial hemorrhage

    Neonatal asphyxia

    Encephalopathy

Brachial plexus injury

Iatrogenic prematurity

Transitional changes

Neonatal infection

Neonatal length of hospital stay

Fetal laceration or trauma

Mother-infant bonding

Long-term outcomes

Fetal mortality

Neonatal mortality

[a] Moderate level evidence.[5]

planned vaginal delivery, 56.7% delivered vaginally and 22% with forceps. The two study groups had no significant differences in overall composite morbidity (planned cesarean versus planned vaginal delivery (relative risk [RR] 1.13, 95% CI 0.92–1.39) or specific outcomes of hemorrhage, transfusion, genital tract injury, wound complications, systemic infection, or depression.[8,9] There were no hysterectomies or cases of thromboembolism and, although pain with planned cesarean was more frequently abdominal rather than genital, no significant differences in rates of pain or depression were appreciated at 3-month follow-up.

A Cochrane Database Systematic Review assessed short-term maternal outcomes of three randomized trials comparing planned cesarean with planned vaginal delivery for breech.[10] The review noted a somewhat increased overall maternal morbidity in the planned cesarean group (9.1% versus 8.6%, RR 1.29, 95% CI 1.03–1.61). Two of the three studies were conducted several decades ago and randomized subjects in labor, thus potentially adding to operative morbidity among cesareans and questioning their applicability to CDMRs today.[7]

Benefits of a vaginal delivery include shorter length of hospital stay and lower rates of infection (eg, endometritis and cystitis).[2] Anesthesia complications are lowest in vaginal deliveries and highest during emergency induction of anesthesia, such as those performed for unplanned, emergent cesareans. Postpartum hemorrhage occurs less frequently in planned cesareans than planned vaginal or unplanned cesareans. However, much of the higher hemorrhage incidence in the planned vaginal delivery group reflects the contribution of operative vaginal deliveries and cesarean in labor.[2] Although a meta-analysis suggests that neonates delivered by cesarean are less likely to initiate breast-feeding, there does not appear to be any difference at 3 or 24 months.[9,11] Maternal mortality, hysterectomy, and thromboembolism are rare outcomes and therefore data on their impact are limited. Lack of data exists for other important variables, such as postpartum pain and depression. Overall, however, the current literature suggests that composite short-term maternal morbidity is similar in women undergoing planned vaginal and planned cesarean deliveries.

Pelvic Floor Dysfunction

The role of cesarean in preventing pelvic floor dysfunction is discussed in detail in Drs. Wohlrab and Rardin's article elsewhere in this issue. Overall, there may be a potential benefit of planned cesareans on short-term stress urinary incontinence. However, this benefit appears to be eliminated in older, parous, and obese patients.[12,13] Cesarean delivery is most protective for urinary incontinence in primiparas women with no urinary incontinence before or during pregnancy.[12]

The literature on anorectal dysfunction, sexual function, and pelvic organ prolapse presents no convincing evidence either favoring cesarean delivery or discouraging it. Anal incontinence following vaginal delivery is strongly associated with overt and occult sphincter lacerations and operative vaginal delivery.[14]

Subsequent Pregnancies

One of the biggest concerns about cesarean delivery is its potential impact on a woman's future reproductive health. Cesareans represent a well-established risk factor for subsequent development of abnormal placentation, including placenta previa and accreta. Although the exact mechanism is unknown, it is commonly hypothesized that uterine scarring prevents normal implantation and migration of the placenta. A large meta-analysis by Faiz and Ananth[2,15] examining the relationship between previa and a history of cesarean deliveries was recently updated for the NIH conference. In a review of 34 studies from 1966 to 2005, the adjusted odds ratio for placenta previa relative to one or more prior cesarean deliveries was 1.32 (95% CI 1.04–1.68) for those studies considered well designed by the investigators and 4.7 (95% CI 1.9–11.4) for poorly designed studies.

Previously estimated at 1:2500 deliveries, the incidence of placenta accreta appears to be rising coincident with higher cesarean rates as a recent study reported 1:533 pregnancies complicated by accreta over a 20-year period from 1982 to 2002.[16,17] Although rare, the condition is clinically significant as accreta has become the leading indication for cesarean-hysterectomy in many centers and can lead to massive obstetric hemorrhage with subsequent disseminated intravascular coagulopathy, surgical visceral injury, adult respiratory distress syndrome, renal failure, or death.[18] Placenta accreta occurs most frequently in women with a prior cesarean (Table 1) who have a placenta previa. Studies estimate the risk for placenta accreta to be 11% to 24% in such women.[19–21]

Concern has been expressed that there may be a relationship between prior cesarean delivery and a subsequent pregnancy resulting in stillbirth. Four major studies have demonstrated no consistent relationship with two showing an increased risk and two showing no difference.[22–25] A recent retrospective cohort dataset of 81,784 deliveries showed an adjusted hazard ratio for all stillbirths of 1.58 (95% CI 0.95-2.63) with the risk mainly concentrated in a subgroup of explained stillbirths.[22] Alternatively, Bahtiyar and colleagues[23] performed a cross-sectional study of United States perinatal mortality data (1995–1997) on over 11 million deliveries and found no difference in the risk for term intrauterine fetal death (RR 0.90, 95% CI 0.76–1.06) in women with a previous cesarean section. Conversely, Salihu and colleagues[24] reviewed a 1978 to 1997 Missouri dataset of 396,441 women and concluded that no association exists between stillbirth and previous cesarean delivery overall but black mothers had a 40% higher likelihood for subsequent stillbirth than whites. Finally, Smith and colleagues[25] analyzed linked datasets from 1980 to 1998 of 120,633 births in Scotland and found a risk of unexplained stillbirth in women with a history of cesarean (adjusted hazard ratio 2.23, 95% CI 1.48–3.36). In this well-designed study, the absolute risk of unexplained stillbirth at or after 39 weeks' gestation was 1.1 per 1000 for women who had a previous cesarean and 0.5 per 1000 in those who had not.[25]

Other reproductive consequences from cesarean delivery include increased risks of spontaneous abortion and ectopic pregnancy, infertility, uterine scar dehiscence, uterine rupture, and placental abruption. In addition, an entity rarely seen in the past, cesarean scar ectopic pregnancies have increased in incidence. In a recent review of 112 cases of cesarean scar pregnancies, more than half (52%) had only one prior cesarean.[26]

Table 1
Cesarean deliveries and the risk of abnormal placentation and hysterectomy

Cesarean #	Accreta (%)[21]	Previa (%)[19]	Previa-Accreta (%)		Hysterectomy (%)[21]
			19	20	
Primary	0.24	0.26	5	3	0.65
Second	0.31	0.65	24	11	0.42
Third	0.57	1.8	47	39	0.90
Fourth	2.13	3	40	60	2.41
Fifth	2.33	10	67	—	3.49

Maternal Mortality

Death associated with pregnancy rarely occurs in modern medicine. Therefore, current studies lack adequate power to quantify a relationship between mortality and method of delivery. Lydon-Rochelle and coworkers[27] published a retrospective cohort study on live-born singletons in Washington state between 1987 and 1996 and found the cesarean delivery maternal mortality rate was 10.3 per 100,000 or approximately four times the rate in the vaginal delivery group. After controlling for age alone or age and severe preeclampsia, however, there was no statistically significant difference. The investigators concluded that cesareans could be a marker for serious preexisting morbidities, which are themselves associated with an increased maternal mortality risk, rather than representing a direct risk of death from the procedure.

A study from the United Kingdom emphasizes the difference between cesareans performed electively and those performed unexpectedly or after the onset of labor. The "Report on Confidential Enquiries into Maternal Death, 1997–1999," found the relative risk of death with cesarean statistically insignificant as compared with vaginal delivery but the greatest risk for maternal mortality occurred with emergency cesarean deliveries.[28] In the 2000–2002 report, however, an increased risk of maternal death was cited with scheduled and elective cesareans (RR 2.8, 95% CI 1.9–4.4) as well as with emergency and urgent cesarean deliveries (RR 4.3, 95% CI 3.0–6.3) when compared with vaginal delivery.[29] The investigators emphasized that determining whether maternal death was a direct consequence of the method of delivery or a coincidental occurrence was difficult and that none of the deaths were associated with CDMR or anesthesia complications.

In summary, the current literature suggests that there is not a net increased risk of maternal death with CDMR but the data are inadequate to accurately estimate the absolute risk of maternal mortality with CDMR.

IMPACT ON THE NEONATE
Overview of Neonatal Morbidity

As in the case of maternal outcomes, the literature is limited on neonatal outcomes from CDMRs. Of most concern regarding the impact of CDMR on neonatal outcomes is the potential for increasing the frequency of neonatal respiratory morbidity. Although serious respiratory distress results primarily from iatrogenic prematurity, transient tachypnea of the newborn and persistent pulmonary hypertension are both increased with elective cesarean delivery regardless of gestational age.[30] Therefore, potential benefits for the neonate from vaginal delivery include a lower risk of respiratory problems, less risk of iatrogenic prematurity, and shorter length of hospital stay.

Studies on elective cesarean delivery before labor show an increased rate of nonrespiratory complications related to neonatal adaptation, such as hypothermia, hypoglycemia, and neonatal intensive care unit admissions, but lower risk of sepsis and meconium aspiration syndrome. Conversely, rare but serious complications, such as intracranial hemorrhage, neonatal asphyxia, and hypoxic encephalopathy are more frequently found following complicated vaginal deliveries and unplanned cesareans. Not surprisingly, brachial plexus injury is higher for infants born via the vaginal route as compared with cesarean. Finally, elective cesareans pose a lower risk for fetal lacerations than unscheduled cesareans.

Unexplained stillbirth remains a devastating obstetric problem that could be reduced by elective cesarean performed before labor.[31,32] While elective cesearean at 39 weeks would eliminate late-term stillbirth, studies supporting this approach are limited as are investigations of the impact of CDMR on long-term neonatal outcomes, such as bonding, early behavioral issues, and developmental outcomes.

Respiratory Morbidity

Perhaps the most concerning CDMR issue for neonates is the potential for increased respiratory morbidity. Respiratory distress syndrome requiring mechanical ventilation is significantly reduced to 1 in 10,000 newborns if elective cesarean delivery is delayed until after 39 weeks' gestation.[33] There is insufficient evidence to determine whether gestational age alone accounts for the differential risk of neonatal respiratory morbidity associated with cesarean compared with vaginal delivery or whether other factors are also involved. Nonetheless, studies that account for gestational age find a consistent and significant reduction in this risk as gestational age exceeds 39 weeks.

Morrison and colleagues[33] prospectively evaluated over 33,000 deliveries at term (≥37 weeks' gestation) over 9 years and found that respiratory morbidity was significantly higher for neonates delivered by cesarean before the onset of labor (35.5 per 1000) compared with cesarean during labor (12.2 per 1000) (odds ratio 2.9, 95% CI 1.9–4.4; $P < .001$), and compared with vaginal delivery (5.3 per 1000) (odds ratio, 6.8; 95% CI 5.2–8.9; $P < .0001$). These findings are consistent with the widely held belief that neonatal passage through the birth canal accompanied by exposure to endogenous steroids and catecholamines released in normal labor and delivery improve the neonatal pulmonary transition from amniotic fluid to breathing air.[30]

While studies have demonstrated the increased risk for respiratory distress and neonatal intensive care unit admission in term infants born by cesarean, these diagnoses are more likely to include transient tachypnea, persistent pulmonary hypertension, or hypoxic respiratory failure rather than "hyaline membrane disease." Despite, the general impression that respiratory morbidity in term infants is benign and self-limited requiring limited intervention, some of these neonates become seriously ill and require prolonged oxygen therapy, mechanical ventilation, and extracorporeal membrane oxygenation. Sometimes, though rarely, the infant dies.[30]

Current recommendations advise limiting administration of corticosteroids to enhance fetal lung maturation to gestations between 24 and 34 weeks.[34] However, at least one study suggests corticosteroid administration in the term gestation may be beneficial. In the Antenatal Steroids for Term Elective Caesarean Section (ASTECS) trial, 998 patients were randomized to steroid administration or no medication before elective cesarean at term (at or after 37 weeks).[35] The incidence of admission with respiratory distress was reduced from 0.051 in the control group and 0.024 in the treatment group (RR 0.46, 95% CI 0.23–0.93).[35] While the findings raise questions about the role antenatal steroids could play in the growing CDMR debate, more studies are needed.

Brachial Plexus Injury, Fetal Trauma, and Neonatal Encephalopathy

Adopting a universal approach of cesarean delivery on all women at 39 weeks has the potential, according to some epidemiologic models, of substantially reducing both transient and permanent brachial plexus injury, neonatal encephalopathy, intrapartum death, and intrauterine fetal demise. Using a hypothetical model assuming a composite estimate for brachial plexus injury risk at 0.15% for vaginal deliveries and applying it to the 3 million deliveries in the United States 39 weeks' gestational age or later, approximately 4500 brachial plexus injuries and 675 (15%) permanent brachial plexus palsies would be avoided if all women underwent cesareans.[36]

Epidemiologic studies suggest that intrapartum hypoxia may be responsible for approximately 10% of cases of neonatal encephalopathy.[37] (see the article by Drs. Miller and Depp elsewhere in this issue. In a Western Australian case-control study of 164 term infants with moderate or severe newborn encephalopathy, a decreased risk of neonatal encephalopathy was observed with elective cesarean compared with spontaneous vaginal delivery (adjusted odds ratio 0.17, 95% CI 0.05–0.56).[38] In this study, Badawi and colleagues[38,39] found the prevalence of encephalopathy to be 3.8 per 1000 for term live births. Antepartum risk factors alone were identified in 69% of affected infants, the cause was unknown in 2%, intrapartum hypoxia in isolation accounted for 4%, and both antepartum risk factors combined with intrapartum hypoxia may have accounted for another 25% of the injuries. In patients who underwent elective cesarean without labor, there was an 83% reduction in the risk of moderate or severe neonatal encephalopathy. This hypothetically amounts to approximately 5000 elective cesareans to prevent 1 case of hypoxic ischemic encephalopathy.[36]

Intrauterine Fetal Death

Stillbirths occur in nearly 1% (6.4 per 1000) of all births in the United States, a rate that equals the mortality due to prematurity and sudden infant death syndrome combined.[40] Particularly problematic is the fact that a substantial number of cases are unexplained. Delivery at 39 weeks would eliminate approximately 6000 stillbirths per year, an intervention that would surpass any prior strategy implemented for stillbirth reduction in regards to efficacy.[36] However, when considering this policy, one must weigh the prospective risk of fetal death, with the risk of neonatal morbidity and mortality exposed at birth.[31]

The balance between averting fetal death and inducing prematurity is a constant obstetric dilemma. Delivery at a given gestational age undoubtedly averts the risk of stillbirth but there has been some recent concern that this approach has contributed to a rise in the number of births between 34 and 37 weeks' gestation, exposing a large number of neonates to complications of late-preterm birth.[41] Barros and colleagues[42] analyzed a prospective cohort of all urban births in Brazil in 1982, 1993, and 2004. The prevalence of preterm births increased from 6.3% to 16.2%, and the rate of cesareans increased from 28% to 43% with cesarean birth performed for 82% of all private deliveries in 2004. The investigators concluded that "excessive medicalization including labor induction, cesareans, and inaccurate ultrasound scans—led by an unregulated private sector with spill-over effects to the public sector, might offset the gains resulting from improved maternal health and newborn survival."[42] The experience in Brazil, a country where cesarean rates supersede those of the United States, cautions of a slippery slope where acknowledging maternal request as an indication for cesarean may open the door for iatrogenic late-preterm births.

PATIENT AND PHYSICIAN ATTITUDES

Despite the best attempts at informed consent and a mutually respectful relationship between providers and their patients, obstetricians and expectant mothers may have different understandings of these two delivery processes. In a 2003 telephone survey of 301 female members of the American College of Obstetricians and Gynecologists (ACOG), 78% of women obstetricians reported having at least one pregnancy and, of those physicians, 27% reported at least one cesarean, of which 22% were elective.[43] Women obstetricians under 40 years old were the most likely age group (41%) to say they would not do a CDMR. In addition to age and gender, other factors, such as career experience and subspecialty, may influence an individual's perspective.

Wu and colleagues[44] used a Web-based questionnaire to survey 782 members of the American Urogynecologic Society (AUGS) and the Society for Maternal-Fetal Medicine (SMFM). Over 45% of AUGS respondents stated that they would choose a cesarean delivery for themselves or their partner for their first pregnancy compared with 9.5% of SMFM members ($P < .001$). In a logistic regression model accounting for each member's age, sex, years in practice, subspecialty, and whether or not the member had children, AUGS members were more likely than SMFM members to agree to perform an elective cesarean (odds ratio 3.4, 95% CI 2.3–4.9, $P < .001$).[44]

Most obstetrician-gynecologists recognize an increased demand for CDMRs within their practices and agree that evidence regarding risks and benefits is crucial to guiding decision-making. A 2006 survey asking ACOG members about their knowledge, perception, and practice patterns regarding CDMR found that 54.6% believed women have the right to a CDMR but 92.2% did not have a policy regarding the procedure.[45] Respondents attributed the increase in inquiries to the increase in information from the media and to convenience and cited more risks than benefits of CDMR. Although women were generally more negative than their male colleagues, there was no relationship between risk/benefit assessment or practice with clinician age or patient characteristics. Finally, Pevzner and colleagues[46] recently explored patient attitudes related to CDMR in an urban setting. Out of 188 written responses, 95% of patients did not believe that CDMR was advisable with the most common explanations classified into categories of "normal is better" or "risk of complications." However, as the investigators acknowledge, most patients studied were members of minorities and, therefore, exploring these questions in other patient populations may yield different results. Patient ethnicity, socioeconomic status, cultural background, and expectations influence attitudes regarding childbirth and more studies are needed addressing patient preferences and attitudes toward CDMR.

AN ETHICAL QUESTION

The paradigm shift and confusion that has surrounded cesarean deliveries is reflected in the terminology found in existing literature. Do these surgeries represent patient choice, patient demand, or patient request?[47] While they refer to the same technical procedure, the ethics and thoughts behind each differ. The final verdict regarding CDMRs remains unanswered. Major organizations, including ACOG and International Federation of Obstetrics and Gynecology have published opinions stating that performing these surgeries is consistent with ethical principles under some circumstances and inconsistent with ethical principles under other circumstances.[5,48,49] When discussing the impact of CDMR on mother and neonate, there are a number of talking points to keep in mind when counseling patients (**Box 2**). After completing the process of informed consent, if personal bias or beliefs hinder the provider from executing the patient's wishes, then referral to another practitioner is advised.[5,49] Although second opinions should be liberally sought when patient uncertainty exists, a recent randomized study in Latin America demonstrated that mandatory second opinions eliminated only 7.3% of cesarean deliveries.[50]

Advantages and adverse outcomes from CDMRs also exist for the obstetrician. Proponents of vaginal deliveries have argued that there is too much technology and intervention in childbirth and that these elective surgeries represent yet another form of birth medicalization. Providers may be hesitant to document CDMRs because of fear of insurance coverage refusal or medical-legal concerns. Others may decline performing them because of personal feelings or beliefs. Obstetricians are often accused of practicing defensive medicine despite studies that have failed to consistently demonstrate that

---

Box 2
Talking points for informed consent on CDMR

- Do not recommend or offer CDMR.
- When a patient solicits a CDMR, inquire the reasons why, educate, and address misconceptions.
- Complete the informed consent process in a nonstressful environment.
- Contemporaneous documentation is ideal.
- Use the intent-to-treat approach and acknowledge that several outcomes exist for planned vaginal or cesarean delivery.
- Be explicit in discussing the known risks, benefits, and alternatives.
- Discuss risks to future pregnancies, including abnormal placentation and uterine rupture.
- Adhere to general ACOG guidelines regarding the timing of elective delivery at or later than 39 weeks' gestation or after documented fetal lung injury.
- After informed consent, if a physician disagrees or is unable to acquiesce to the patient's decision, refer to another health care provider.

---

medical-legal experiences significantly affect the health care delivery.[51] Accountability in health care remains a reality, however, and 76% of obstetricians surveyed in 2003 reported a litigation event at some point in their careers, most often for allegedly causing cerebral palsy, a condition that cannot be eradicated by cesarean delivery.[37,52]

Because of the complexity of this question, the decision-making approach required to process and deliberate all aspects of this may vary for each individual. In addition to the medical impact, discussions should also include psychologic, economic, and sociologic considerations and may focus on mental and behavioral characteristics, probabilities and finances, or societal implications.[53] All these viewpoints are valid and obstetricians have a responsibility to their patients to incorporate all these considerations. Of female ACOG members surveyed, 32% (and depending on circumstances, an additional 28%) would acquiesce to their patient's request for an elective cesarean.[43] Patients with reservations are more likely to have greater concerns with regard to maternal and fetal risks, suggesting that a more detailed risk disclosure before the procedure is warranted for all pregnant patients to prevent physician-patient conflict in the intrapartum period.[54] The provider should not be hindered by the reality of a busy practice and managed care and must see that the process of informed consent is complete and documented. He or she is left with the burden to prove that the components of informed consent are executed properly and fully. Above all, patient autonomy must be maintained. Exercising this cooperative decision-making process is a delicate balance but part of the altruistic privilege of being a physician.[55] Only by listening and skillful ommunication can we empower patients with autonomy.

SUMMARY

No systematic, well-designed data exist on CDMR. However the rate of primary cesareans is increasing and studies using hospital discharge data or birth certificate data estimate that from 3% to 7% of all deliveries to women without prior cesareans have no reported medical or obstetric indication for their primary cesarean deliveries.[2] The absolute risk of neonatal and maternal morbidity is small with either cesarean or vaginal delivery. Mothers are often willing to take the burden of risk to optimize outcome for their unborn child, but should be counseled that the most concerning risks affect the mother's future reproduction with life-threatening conditions, such as placenta accreta. Counseling mothers on the potential risks and benefits has become more challenging as there has been growing interest without a simultaneous cohesive effort to learn more about this procedure. As our views about the birth process change, there will certainly be a palpable impact of the rising cesarean rate for providers, hospitals, and parents.

The literature suggests that overall risks of maternal complications with elective cesarean are slightly lower than a trial of vaginal delivery and are primarily driven by the incidence of cesarean delivery occurring during labor and its associated increased rate of complications. This stresses the importance of an intent-to-treat approach for future research.

When addressing risks and benefits with patients, there are three areas of importance. First, the risk for abnormal placentation with future pregnancies should be emphasized. According to the latest US Census, 67% of women at the end of the reproductive age range have two or more children.[56] Because many women have several children and because prior cesarean is an important and known risk factor for placenta previa and accreta, implications to future childbearing should always be mentioned. Secondly, there are many areas on which studies are lacking. All studies reviewed in the NICHD conference included proxy comparison groups. Caution must be taken when interpreting existing studies, as there are no current optimal studies comparing the optimal groups of planned vaginal delivery to CDMR. Recent surveys of both laypersons and obstetricians reveal that a substantial number (27%) of women cite fear of the act of childbirth itself to justify their chosen delivery route.[57,58] Eliciting the patient's specific fears or concerns is therefore an important step in correcting misconceptions and alleviating irrational fears. Finally, numerous factors that can alter the risks and benefits—such as culture, maternal obesity, and provider background—must be acknowledged.

A survey of the literature published since the 2006 NIH state-of-the-science conference reveals many editorials, commentaries, and review articles but few original studies on CDMR. Studies from investigators both in the United States and from such countries as China have found that the rate of CDMRs have increased dramatically in recent years.[59,60] However, these studies are largely population based and their limitations include those related to the reliability and accuracy of the data, such as, for example, data from discharge surveys, and extrapolations made to CDMR. Even those reviews that are thorough must acknowledge that the evidence is significantly limited by its relevance to primary CDMR.[61] In summary, recently published research has been informative and successful in focusing attention on CDMR but has been disappointing in both the quality and quantity of studies needed.

Until more rigorous information is gathered about CDMRs and until practice standards and guidelines are implemented, an explicitly executed informed consent should form the framework of any decision regarding mode of delivery. Some have expressed concern of how well women can be counseled regarding the birth process and how well they are able to truly understand and incorporate future sequelae into the decision-making process. However, we are reminded that each individual is the best proponent for his or her own welfare and each expectant mother is the best advocate for the health of her unborn child.

REFERENCES

1. Hamilton BE, Martin JA, Ventura SJ. Births: preliminary data for 2006. Natl Vital Stat Rep 2007;56(7):1–18.

2. National Institutes of Health state-of-the-science conference statement. Cesarean delivery on maternal request. March 27–29, 2006. Obstet Gynecol 2006;107: 1386–97.
3. Wittekindt C, Kribs A, Roth B, et al. Rupture of the larynx in a newborn. Obstet Gynecol 2002;99(5 Pt 2):904–6.
4. Kaluarachchi A, Krishnamurthy S. Post–cesarean section splenic rupture. Am J Obstet Gynecol 1995;173(1):230–2.
5. American College of Obstetricians and Gynecologists. Cesarean delivery on maternal request. ACOG Committee Opinion No. 394. Obstet Gynecol 2007;110: 1501–4.
6. Minkoff H, Chervenak FA. Elective primary cesarean delivery. N Engl J Med 2003; 348(10):946–50.
7. Wax JR. Maternal request cesarean versus planned spontaneous vaginal delivery: maternal morbidity and short term outcomes. Semin Perinatol 2006;30: 247–52.
8. Hannah ME, Hannah WJ, Hewson SA, et al. Planned caesarean section versus planned vaginal birth for breech presentation at term: a randomised multicentre trial. Lancet 2000;356:1375–83.
9. Hannah ME, Hannah WJ, Hodnett ED, et al. Outcomes at 3 months after planned cesarean vs. planned vaginal delivery for breech presentation at term. J Am Med Assoc 2002;287:1822–31.
10. Hofmeyr GJ, Hannah ME. Planned cesarean section for term breech delivery. Cochrane Database Syst Rev 2003;3:CD000166.
11. Hannah ME, Whyte H, Hannah WJ, et al. Maternal outcomes at 2 years after planned cesarean section versus planned vaginal birth for breech presentation at term: the international randomized Term Breech Trial. Term Breech Trial Collaborative Group. Am J Obstet Gynecol 2004;191:917–27.
12. Nygaard I. Urinary incontinence: Is cesarean delivery protective? Semin Perinatol 2006;30:267–71.
13. Rortveit G, Hannestad YS, Daltveit AK, et al. Age and type-dependent effects of parity on urinary incontinence: the Norwegian EPINCONT study. Obstet Gynecol 2001;98:1004–10.
14. Eason E, Labrecque M, Marcoux S, et al. Anal incontinence after childbirth. CMAJ 2002;166:326–30.
15. Faiz AS, Ananth CV. Etiology and risk factors for placenta previa: an overview and meta-analysis of observational studies. J Matern Fetal Neonatal Med 2003;13(3): 175–90.
16. Miller DA, Chollet JA, Goodwin TM. Clinical risk factors for placenta previa-placenta accreta. Am J Obstet Gynecol 1997;177:210–4.
17. Wu S, Kocherginsky M, Hibbard JU. Abnormal placentations: twenty-year analysis. Am J Obstet Gynecol 2005;192:1458–61.
18. Oyelese Y, Smulian JC. Placenta previa, placenta accreta, and vasa previa. Obstet Gynecol 2006;107:927–41.
19. Clark SL, Koonings PP, Phelan JP. Placenta previa / accreta and prior cesarean section. Obstet Gynecol 1985;66:89–92.
20. Grobman WA, Gersnoviez R, Landon MB, et al. Pregnancy outcomes for women with placenta previa in relation to the number of prior cesarean deliveries. Obstet Gynecol 2007;110:1249–55.
21. Silver RM, Landon MB, Rouse DJ, et al. Maternal morbidity associated with multiple repeat cesarean deliveries. NICHD-MFMU Network. Obstet Gynecol 2006; 107:1226–32.

22. Gray R, Quigley MA, Hockley C, et al. Caesarean delivery and risk of stillbirth in subsequent pregnancy: a retrospective cohort study in an English population. BJOG 2007;114(3):264–70.
23. Bahtiyar MO, Julien S, Robinson JN, et al. Prior cesarean delivery is not associated with an increased risk of stillbirth in a subsequent pregnancy: analysis of U.S. perinatal mortality data, 1995–1997. Am J Obstet Gynecol 2006;195(5): 1373–8.
24. Salihu HM, Sharma PP, Kristensen S, et al. Risk of stillbirth following a cesarean delivery: black-white disparity. Obstet Gynecol 2006;107(2 Pt 1):383–90.
25. Smith G, Pell JP, Dobbie R. Caesarean section and risk of unexplained stillbirth in subsequent pregnancy. Lancet 2003;362(9398):1779–84.
26. Rotas MA, Haberman S, Levgur M. Cesarean scar ectopic pregnancies: etiology, diagnosis, and management. Obstet Gynecol 2006;107:1373–81.
27. Lydon-Rochelle M, Holy VL, Easterling TR. Cesarean delivery and postpartum mortality among primiparas in Washington state, 1987–1996. Obstet Gynecol 2001;97:169 74.
28. Department of Health, Scottish Executive Health Department, Department of Health, Social Services, and Public Safety, Northern Ireland. Why mothers die. Fifth report on confidential enquiries into maternal deaths in the United Kingdom, 1997–1999. London: RCOG Press; 2001.
29. Department of Health, Scottish Executive Health Department, Department of Health, Social Services, and Public Safety, Northern Ireland. Why mothers die. Fifth report on confidential enquiries into maternal deaths in the United Kingdom, 2000–2002. London: RCOG Press; 2004.
30. Jain L, Dudell GG. Respiratory transition in infants delivered by cesarean section. Semin Perinatol 2006;30:296 304.
31. Kahn B, Lumey LH, Zybert PA, et al. Prospective risk of fetal death in singleton, twin, and triplet gestations: implications for practice. Obstet Gynecol 2003;102: 685–92.
32. Reddy UM. Prediction and prevention of recurrent stillbirth. Obstet Gynecol 2007; 110:1151–64.
33. Morrison JJ, Rennie JM, Milton PJ. Neonatal respiratory morbidity and mode of delivery at term: influence of timing of elective caesarean section. Br J Obstet Gynaecol 1995;102:101–6.
34. American College of Obstetricians and Gynecologists. Antenatal corticosteroid therapy for fetal maturation. ACOG Committee Opinion No. 273. Obstet Gynecol 2008;111:805–7.
35. Stutchfield P, Whitaker R, Russell I, et al. Antenatal betamethasone and incidence of neonatal respiratory distress after elective caesarean section: pragmatic randomized trial. BMJ 2005;331:662–8.
36. Hankins GD, Clark SM, Munn MB. Cesarean section on request at 39 weeks: impact on shoulder dystocia, fetal trauma, neonatal encephalopathy, and intrauterine fetal demise. Semin Perinatol 2006;30:276–87.
37. American College of Obstetricians and Gynecologists, American Academy of Pediatrics. Neonatal encephalopathy and cerebral palsy: defining the pathogenesis and pathophysiology. Washington, DC: ACOG and AAP; 2003.
38. Badawi N, Kurinczuk JJ, Keogh JM, et al. Antepartum risk factors for newborn encephalopathy: the Western Australian case-control study. BMJ 1998;317: 1549–53.
39. Badawi N, Kurinczuk JJ, Keogh JM, et al. Intrapartum risk factors for newborn encephalopathy: the Western Australian case-control study. BMJ 1998;317:1554–8.

40. Silver RM. Fetal death. Obstet Gynecol 2007;109:153–67.
41. Raju TN, Higgins RD, Stark AR, et al. Optimizing care and outcome for late pre-term (near-term) infants: a summary of the workshop sponsored by the NICHD. Pediatrics 2006;118(3):1207–14.
42. Barros FC, Victora CG, Barros AJ, et al. The challenge of reducing neonatal mortality in middle-income countries: findings from three Brazilian birth cohorts in 1982, 1993, and 2004. Lancet 2005;365(9462):847–54.
43. American College of Obstetricians and Gynecologists. ACOG unveils survey of women ob-gyns at media briefing. ACOG Today. 2004; volume 48:2.
44. Wu JM, Hundley AF, Visco AG. Elective primary cesarean delivery: attitudes of urogynecology and maternal-fetal medicine specialists. Obstet Gynecol 2005; 105(2):301–6.
45. Bettes BA, Coleman VH, Zinberg S, et al. Cesarean delivery on maternal request: obstetrician-gynecologist's knowledge, perception, and practice patterns. Obstet Gynecol 2007;109(1):57–66.
46. Pevzner L, Goffman D, Freda MC, et al. Patients' attitudes associated with cesarean delivery on maternal request in an urban population. Am J Obstet Gynecol 2008;198(5):e35–7.
47. Lee YM, D'Alton ME. Cesarean delivery: a choice, a demand, or a request? Ann Fam Med 2006;4:265–8.
48. FIGO Committee for the Ethical Aspect of Human Reproduction and Women's Health. Int J Gynaecol Obstet 1999;64:317–22.
49. American College of Obstetricians and Gynecologists. Surgery and patient choice. ACOG Committee Opinion No. 395. Obstet Gynecol 2008;111:243–7.
50. Althabe F, Belizan JM, Villar J, et al. Mandatory second opinion to reduce rates of unnecessary caesarean sections in Latin America: a cluster randomised controlled trial. Lancet 2004;363:1934–40.
51. Baicker K, Chandra A. The effect of malpractice liability on the delivery of health care. NBER Working Paper. National Bureau of Economic Research Conference Frontiers in Health Policy June 24, 2004.
52. Hankins GD, MacLennan AH, Speer ME, et al. Obstetric litigation is asphyxiating our maternity services. Obstet Gynecol 2006;107(6):1382–5.
53. Minkoff H. The ethics of cesarean section by choice. Semin Perinatol 2006;30: 309–12.
54. Lescale KB, Inglis SR, Eddleman KA, et al. Conflicts between physicians and patients in non-elective cesarean delivery: incidence and the adequacy of informed consent. Am J Perinatol 1996;13(3):171–6.
55. Eisenberg C. It is still a privilege to be a doctor. N Engl J Med 1986;314(17): 1113–4.
56. US Census Bureau. Fertility of American women. June 2004;Issued December 2005.
57. Wax JR, Cartin A, Pinette MG, et al. Patient choice cesarean: an evidence-based review. Obstet Gynecol Surv 2004;59(8):601–16.
58. Wax JR, Cartin A, Pinette MG, et al. Patient choice cesarean—the Maine experience. Birth 2005;32(3):203–6.
59. Gossman GL, Joesch JM, Tanfer K. Trends in maternal request cesarean delivery from 1991 to 2004. Obstet Gynecol 2006;108:1506–16.
60. Zhang J, Liu Y, Meikle S, et al. Cesarean delivery on maternal request in southeast China. Obstet Gynecol 2008;111(5):1077–82.
61. Visco AG, Viswanathan M, Lohr KH, et al. Cesarean delivery on maternal request: maternal and neonatal outcomes. Obstet Gynecol 2006;108(6):1517–29.

Placenta Accreta and Cesarean Scar Pregnancy: Overlooked Costs of the Rising Cesarean Section Rate

Todd Rosen, MD

KEYWORDS

- Abnormal placental implantation • Placenta accreta
- Cesarean scar ectopic pregnancies

The cesarean delivery rate in the United States rose to 31.1% of all births in 2006,[1] an increase over the 2005 rate and another consecutive record high. The percentage of all births delivered by cesarean section has climbed 50% over the last decade from a nadir of 20.7% in 1996. Although the risks to women during the current pregnancy from cesarean section may not be excessive when compared with those associated with vaginal delivery, the risks to subsequent pregnancies are not given enough consideration in the risk-benefit calculus when determining the route of delivery. For example, family size may be limited by the increasing risks of repetitive cesarean sections. In addition, the risk for antenatal stillbirth may be increased in women with a prior cesarean section when compared with women with prior vaginal births.[2] Perhaps the greatest risk to future pregnancies is an increase in disorders caused by abnormal placentation, including placenta accreta and cesarean section scar ectopic pregnancies. The focus of this review is to describe how uterine scarring from cesarean section may lead to these serious disorders and how to diagnose and manage these problems.

CESAREAN SECTION LEADS TO ABNORMAL PLACENTAL IMPLANTATION

The placenta begins to form between days 13 and 15 after ovulation, and, initially during the embryonic period, chorionic villi composed of trophoblast cells cover the entire surface of the gestational sac. As the fetal period begins, the villi overlying the decidua capsularis degenerate to form the chorion laeve, while the villi over the decidua basalis proliferate to form the definitive placenta.[3]

Division of Maternal-Fetal Medicine, Department of Obstetrics and Gynecology, 622 West 168th Street, PH 16-66, Columbia University, New York, NY 10032, USA
E-mail address: tr2171@columbia.edu

Clin Perinatol 35 (2008) 519–529
doi:10.1016/j.clp.2008.07.003
0095-5108/08/$ – see front matter © 2008 Elsevier Inc. All rights reserved.

Normal implantation of the placenta is critical to the success of the pregnancy, and this process is tightly regulated. A large number of cytokines, steroid hormones, immunologic factors, prostaglandins, and other mediators are critical to successful placentation.[4] Strong evidence suggests that local oxygen levels have an important role in regulating differentiation and proliferation of the trophoblast. This observation has led to speculation that localized disturbances in oxygen tension in the endometrium and myometrium of a cesarean scar may contribute to abnormalities of placentation.

The early embryo develops in a relatively hypoxic environment. Direct measures of oxygen concentration in the endometrium shows tension levels between 2% and 5%.[5] Initially, invading trophoblast cells plug the lumina of the decidual vessels, further contributing to the physiologic hypoxia. In addition, the basal laminae of proliferating cytotrophoblast is thicker in early pregnancy, slowing oxygen diffusion to the embryo. Not until 10 to 12 weeks of pregnancy does blood flow into the intervillous space begin.

This physiologic hypoxia appears to stimulate the cytotrophoblast cells to undergo mitosis, which is different than most other cell types. Under these conditions, the cytotrophoblast invades the endometrium, reaching the spiral arterioles, and then differentiates into a vascular phenotype.[6] In vitro work demonstrates that oxygen tension determines whether cytotrophoblast cells proliferate or invade, regulating placental growth and architecture.[7] Because the early embryo requires a hypoxic environment, it may preferentially implant into a cesarean section scar, which tends to be acellular and avascular. This tendency may explain the increased risk for placenta previa and accreta in individuals with an increasing number of cesarean sections.[8] Alternatively, the placenta may preferentially develop in a hypoxic scar, not involuting over this area, as it would in an unscarred uterus.

Trophoblast implanting over an avascular scar may invade more deeply into the uterine wall because of the prolonged maintenance of an invasive phenotype. This delay in arrest of mitosis with subsequent initiation of differentiation is likely secondary to the absence of underlying tissue with normal vasculature and high oxygen tension.

PLACENTA ACCRETA

Placenta accreta occurs when the placenta becomes abnormally adherent to the myometrium rather than the uterine decidua (**Fig. 1**). If the placenta invades into the

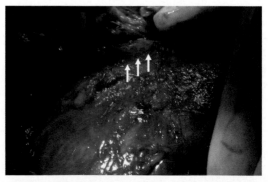

Fig. 1. Intraoperative finding of focal placenta accreta, with an area of placenta abnormally adherent to the myometrium (*arrows*).

myometrium, it is termed *increta*. A placenta *percreta* invades to the level of the serosa or continues into adjacent organs.

Rates of placenta accreta appear to be rising, although the reported incidence varies widely. In a 1977 report, Breen and colleagues[9] found that the incidence in the published literature ranged between 1 in 540 to 1 in 70,000 deliveries. More recently, Miller and colleagues[10] reported an incidence of histologically confirmed placenta accreta of 1 in 2510 for a 10-year period ending in 1994. Over a 20-year period ending in 2002, Wu and colleagues[11] determined an incidence of 1 in 533. The differences most likely reflect methods in case ascertainment. For example, a regional referral center would be expected to have a higher concentration of cases than a general survey across a wide geographic area.

Risk Factors

Risk factors associated with placenta accreta are prior uterine surgery, including cesarean section, uterine curettage, advancing maternal age, and increasing parity. Other associations include prior myomectomy, manual removal of the placenta, prior hysteroscopic surgery, and prior pelvic irradiation. Cases of placenta accreta following endometrial ablation[12] and uterine artery embolization[13] have been reported. Placenta previa is an independent risk factor for concurrent accreta, even in the absence of other risk factors.

Approximately 50% of pregnancies complicated by accreta are preceded by a cesarean delivery in a prior pregnancy.[11] As cesarean rates have continued to rise and the numbers of women with repeat surgeries increase as well, cesarean section will become an even more prevalent antecedent to pregnancies complicated by placenta accreta. In a prospective observational study, the Maternal-Fetal Medicine Units Network evaluated the risk of placenta accreta with increasing numbers of cesarean sections. They found that the risk for placenta accreta was 0.24%, 0.32%, 0.57%, 2.13%, 2.33%, and 6.74% in women undergoing their first, second, third, fourth, fifth, and sixth or more cesarean delivery, respectively.[8] If women were diagnosed with placenta previa, the risk for placenta accreta was 3%, 11%, 40%, 61%, and 67% for the first, second, third, fourth, and fifth or more cesarean section, respectively. The risk for hysterectomy climbed to 2.5% with a woman's fourth cesarean and to 9% with the sixth or more cesarean.

The exact mechanism by which a prior cesarean section predisposes to placenta accreta is uncertain. Traditional teaching has been that, with each cesarean section, the endometrium underlying the implantation site is damaged and becomes unsuitable for subsequent placentation. Subsequent pregnancies are more likely to become implanted in the lower uterine segment by a process of elimination;[14] however, it seems equally likely that, with each successive cesarean section, the uterine scar becomes more accessible to the implanting embryo because successive incisions are created higher in the uterine wall to avoid bladder injury from adhesions or because elective repeat surgeries occur without labor. Whether placenta accreta occurs more frequently following sections not preceded by labor is unknown. Sonographic evaluation of post cesarean uterine scars imaged during subsequent pregnancies demonstrates that surgery performed in labor is more likely to occur in the cervix.[15] Only about half of women whose cesarean sections are performed without labor have a detectable cervical scar, suggesting that the incision is created in the myometrium.

Diagnosis

Antenatal diagnosis of placenta accreta should begin with a high index of suspicion in women having risk factors for this condition. Ultrasound is the most common modality used to make the diagnosis. The sensitivity of ultrasound in detecting placenta accreta in high-risk patients (ie, those with a placenta previa and a history of cesarean section) is approximately 80%, with a specificity of 95%.[16,17] Patients with placental locations away from the lower uterine segment may be more difficult to detect before the time of delivery.

Ultrasound findings typical of placenta accreta and percreta are shown in **Figs. 2** and **3**A. Findings include the absence of a hypolucent area forming a distinct boundary between the placenta and the myometrium, sonolucent lakes of slow flow within the placenta, and increased vascularity demonstrated by color Doppler.[16,18] Hypervascularity of the bladder and uterine serosa may also be observed. In addition, the placenta may appear enlarged or bulky. Diagnosis of placenta accreta is typically made in the second trimester at the time of routine fetal anatomic screening.

Sonographic signs of accreta may be evident in the first trimester. Comstock and colleagues[19] published a retrospective review of ultrasound images before 10 weeks gestational age in women later found to have placenta accreta. Six patients had low-lying gestational sacs, with most appearing to be attached to the uterine scar with thinning of the myometrium. In early gestation, distinguishing a pregnancy likely to become an accreta from a cesarean scar ectopic pregnancy may be difficult. Although in a "scar gestation," the gestational sac is usually not contained within the uterine cavity, absolute distinctions are likely artificial, and these two entities more likely form a continuum with overlap in outcome and clinical management.

MRI may be a useful adjunct in the diagnosis of accreta (**Fig. 3**B, C). Although not used as a screening tool, it may be helpful in cases with inconclusive ultrasound findings. Moreover, it appears to be a better test for determining the extent of myometrial invasion.[20] Warshak and colleagues[16] found that when MRI was performed following a suspicious or inconclusive ultrasound, sensitivity increased from 77% to 88% and specificity from 96% to 100%.

Biologic markers have the potential to further improve the diagnostic accuracy of placenta accreta. Elevated levels of maternal serum creatinine kinase,[21] alpha fetoprotein, and β-human chorionic gonadotropin (βhCG)[22] have been reported in affected pregnancies. Mazouni and colleagues[23] have proposed that assessment of maternal blood for cell-free fetal DNA, placental mRNA, and the use of DNA microarray for placental-specific genes may be useful tools, but data do not yet exist to determine whether they will be useful clinically.

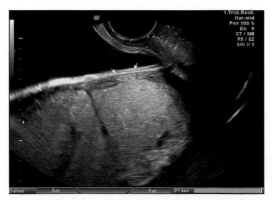

Fig. 2. A discrete area of abnormal invasion of the placenta into the myometrium (*arrows*) in a patient with two prior cesarean sections and placenta previa. There is loss of the normal hypoechoic rim of myometrial tissue beneath the placenta.

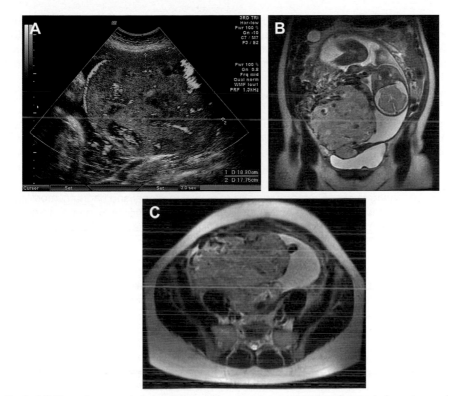

Fig. 3. (A) Placenta percreta in a patient with one prior cesarean section and placenta previa. A bulky heterogenous placenta with multiple venous lakes with flow is demonstrated by power Doppler study. (B) Coronal T2-weighted MRI images of the same placenta percreta in (A). There is marked heterogeneity of signal intensity within the placenta, typical of placenta accreta. The placenta bulges anteriorly into the bladder, distorting the normal uterine architecture. The placenta can be seen invading laterally through the myometrium into the right pelvic side wall in both views. MRI delineates the extent of invasion more accurately than ultrasound. (C) Axial T2-weighted MRI images of the same placenta percreta in (A), again showing marked heterogeneity of signal intensity within the placenta, typical of placenta accreta, and bulging into the bladder.

Delivery Complications

Significant hemorrhage and severe maternal morbidity at the time of delivery are common in cases of placenta accreta. The bleeding may become massive in cases of placenta percreta. Infection, bladder injury, ureteral ligation or fistula formation, and spontaneous uterine rupture are well-known complications of an abnormally invasive placenta.

At the author's center, 33 women were treated with either placenta accreta or percreta confirmed by histopathology between 2001 and 2006. Approximately 50% of these cases were recognized before delivery. None were treated conservatively, and all had hysterectomy. Estimated blood loss during surgery ranged between 2500 and 5000 mL, with an average of 3000 mL. On average, women received 10 units of packed red blood cells, with a range of 3 to 29 units. Admission to the ICU was required for 51.6% of women and 29% had intraoperative complications. Almost 40% had postpartum complications.

O'Brien and colleagues[24] published survey data on outcomes following placenta percreta. Only half of the cases were suspected antepartum. Forty percent of the patients required transfusion with more than 10 units of packed red blood cells; ureteral ligation or fistula formation complicated 10% of cases; infection affected 31%; and perinatal death occurred in 9%. Maternal death occurred in 7% of cases.

Management

Basic principles in the approach to the patient with placenta accreta are outlined herein. Because of the severe morbidity and the potential for maternal death, careful planning to reduce morbidity is essential.

Although guidelines for the management of these complicated cases are limited, a multidisciplinary approach to a suspected placenta accreta or percreta should maximize the management of hemorrhage and minimize maternal and neonatal morbidity. This team may include obstetricians and maternal fetal specialists, gynecologic oncologists or other surgeons with expertise in extensive pelvic surgery, obstetric anesthesia, interventional radiology, and representatives from the blood bank and operating room. At the author's center, all cases of suspected placenta accreta are seen by critical care obstetrics or maternal fetal medicine specialists before surgery and are counseled about the possible clinical outcomes. The appropriate delivery venue and timing for delivery are determined in consultation with the surgical support team, the operating room staff, and obstetric anesthesia. When clinical suspicion is high, delivery is generally performed at 36 weeks gestational age without amniocentesis because of the low risk to the fetus compared with the potential major maternal complications of emergency delivery without appropriate resources in place.

The surgical approach is almost always through a vertical skin incision regardless of any previous scar. An expert pelvic surgeon, often a gynecologic oncologist, should be present from the outset of surgery. Adequate volumes of packed red blood cells (20 units), platelets (12 units), fresh frozen plasma (20 units), and clotting factors are prepared before surgery. Cell saver technology can be safely used during a cesarean section and is frequently employed. In select cases of placenta percreta, interventional radiology and a vascular surgery team are consulted before surgery, and prophylactic arterial embolization or aortic dissection may follow delivery of the fetus before initiation of hysterectomy. Topical hemostatic agents, which are often used during liver surgery, are available before the operation is started. Activated factor VII may be employed to treat postpartum hemorrhage.[25]

In some cases, despite extensive planning and expertise, hemorrhage cannot be controlled intraoperatively. In such cases, the abdomen can be packed to control bleeding and allow time for adequate transfusion of volume, red blood cells, and clotting factors, as well as correction of metabolic acidosis. We prepare an umbrella pack[26] before surgery in the event that this maneuver is required. Following this treatment, the fascia is temporarily closed with towel clamps, the subcutaneous tissue dressed with moist pads, and the patient transferred to the ICU with a plan to return to the operating room after she has been stabilized. Active communication between the operating and anesthesia teams during the entire surgery is essential so that all are aware of the patient's status and can rapidly react when necessary.

Because of the severe morbidity involved with surgical management, especially when cases of placenta accreta or percreta are diagnosed intraoperatively, "conservative" approaches in which the placenta is left in situ are becoming more common. Timmermans and colleagues[27] reviewed 60 cases of abnormally invasive placentation managed by leaving the placenta in situ without hysterectomy. Twenty-six women were managed without any additional interventions. In most of these patients

(19/26), the placenta had been partially removed. In 4 of these 26, conservative ther-apy failed. Twenty-two women received adjuvant methotrexate. In most of these women (19/22), the entire placenta was left in situ. In five, therapy failed. Twelve women were managed with arterial embolization. In most of these patients (9/12), the diagnosis was made antepartum and the placenta was completely left in situ. In three patients, therapy failed. Overall, 11 women experienced infection (11/60), 21 women experienced vaginal bleeding (21/60), and 4 experienced disseminated intravascular coagulopathy (4/60). Spontaneous loss of placental tissue was noted in 16 women. Subsequent pregnancies were reported in eight women. It was con-cluded that conservative management of abnormally invasive placentation can be effective and fertility can be preserved, but it should only be considered in highly selected cases when blood loss is minimal and there is desire for fertility preservation. Whether adjuvant methotrexate or selective arterial embolization is beneficial is uncer-tain. Undetectable hCG values do not seem to guarantee complete resorption of retained placental tissue.

CESAREAN SCAR ECTOPIC PREGNANCIES

The first case of a pregnancy implanted into a cesarean scar was reported in 1978.[28] As of 2006, there were 161 instances reported in either case reports or case series.[29] The frequency of this condition is uncertain and depends on several factors, including the use of routine first-trimester ultrasound. Two recent studies have estimated an incidence of approximately 1 in 2000 pregnancies.[30,31]

As is true for placenta accreta, the exact cause of implantation of the gestation into the scar of a previous cesearean section is not well understood. Investigators have speculated that cesarean scar pregnancies result from implantation through a micro-scopic fistula between the endometrial cavity and the scar;[32] however, as described previously, because the early placenta is an invasive organ capable of digesting extra-cellular matrix proteins, a preexisting tract would not be necessary.

It is reasonable to suppose that the pathologic mechanisms of placenta accreta and scar pregnancies are similar with the site and level of invasion being different. With placenta accreta, the placenta is abnormally adherent to the myometrium with the gestational sac growing into the lumen of the uterus. A cesarean scar ectopic preg-nancy is implanted entirely within the cesarean scar and is surrounded by myometrium and fibrous tissue.[29] It is possible that some placenta accretas and especially percre-tas began as cesarean ectopic pregnancies, with the thickness of the scar and the degree of invasion dictating the subsequent course. Support for a similar pathophys-iology of these two entities comes from reports of cesarean scar ectopic pregnancies diagnosed early in gestation which were managed expectantly, resulting in near-term delivery of a viable neonate.[33] Many of these cases behaved similar to placenta percreta, with massive hemorrhage necessitating hysterectomy. One might also spec-ulate that several case reports of second-trimester and early third-trimester uterine rupture supposedly due to placenta percreta[34,35] would have been diagnosed as cesarean scar pregnancies if early ultrasound had been performed.

Ultrasound Diagnosis of a Cesarean Scar Pregnancy

Jurkovic and colleagues[30] used the following criteria to diagnose early cesarean scar pregnancies by transvaginal sonography (**Fig. 4**):

1. The uterine cavity is empty.
2. The gestational sac is located anteriorly at the level of the internal os, covering the visible or presumed site of the cesarean section scar.

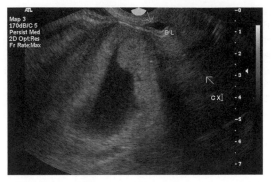

Fig. 4. A midline sagittal image of a cesarean scar pregnancy obtained by transvaginal sonography. The gestational sac is implanted anteriorly between the cervix and an empty uterine cavity. The sac is bulging toward the bladder anteriorly.

3. Doppler study suggests a functional placental circulation defined by increased vascularity by color flow evaluation, a peak velocity greater than 20 cm/s, and a pulsatility index of less than 1.
4. There is no "sliding organs sign," defined as the inability to displace the gestational sac with gentle pressure applied by the transvaginal probe.

MRI[36] and hysteroscopy[37] have been proposed as adjuncts to ultrasound, but at least in early pregnancy, transvaginal ultrasound is an accurate diagnostic tool, and additional modalities are rarely necessary.

Clinical Course and Management of Cesarean Scar Pregnancies

Because most cases of cesarean scar pregnancies identified early in gestation have been terminated, there are insufficient data to adequately quantify the maternal risks of continuing the pregnancy or to predict the likelihood of successfully continuing to viability. Jurkovic and colleagues[30] reported on 18 cesarean scar pregnancies diagnosed in the first trimester of which three were followed expectantly. None of these progressed past 17 weeks, and one woman experienced severe hemorrhage requiring emergency hysterectomy. Because of the potential for severe morbidity associated with this diagnosis, the best medical advice based on current information is for pregnancy termination.

The most effective therapy to terminate a cesarean scar ectopic pregnancy is unknown, and treatment should be individualized. Both medical and surgical approaches have proven successful. Systemic[38] and local injection[36] of methotrexate has been described in published reports. Other agents injected directly into the fetus within a cesarean scar pregnancy have included potassium chloride and hyperosmolar glucose. Surgical sac aspiration[37] has proven successful. Several other surgical approaches, including hysteroscopic,[39] laparascopic,[40] and open removal,[29] have been successfully used.

Uterine curettage has been performed to treat cesarean scar pregnancies, but this approach appears to have a high failure rate. Wang and colleagues[40] reported a failure in 12 of 17 women who underwent uterine curettage as their initial treatment modality.

PREVENTION OF PLACENTA ACCRETA AND CESAREAN SCAR PREGNANCIES

Many placenta accretas and all cesarean scar pregnancies occur following a previous cesarean delivery. The obvious approach to reduce the incidence of these two entities is to reduce the primary cesarean section rate and to revisit the idea of vaginal birth after a first cesarean. At the very least, women considering elective cesarean section should be aware that they may be putting their next pregnancy at increased risk for a potentially devastating complication.

Future studies are needed to evaluate whether surgical techniques are available to reduce the likelihood of a subsequent abnormal placental implantation. Perhaps, modification of the approach to uterine closure may be beneficial, or administration of biologic agents to improve healing and revascularization of the cesarean scar could be effective. It is not known whether a single-layer closure or two-layer closure is more likely to result in accretas or scar pregnancies in subsequent pregnancies. Similarly, many surgeons close the uterus with a running locked suture that is more likely to lead to necrosis and fibrosis at the incision site. It is theoretically possible that avoidance of the locking technique could reduce abnormal placental implantation, and future studies should evaluate this approach.

Delaying cesarean section until the cervix has effaced and the lower segment is developed would make it more likely that the uterine incision is made in the cervix rather than in the isthmus of the uterus. Although some surgeons advocate performing cesarean section without creating a bladder flap, it may be beneficial to dissect the bladder as inferiorly as possible so that the uterine incision can be made in the cervix. Both of these measures have the potential to "hide" the scar from the implanting embryo in subsequent pregnancies, reducing the risk of abnormally invasive placentation.

Early transvaginal ultrasound in all women with prior cesarean sections should be considered to screen for developing placenta accretas or cesarean scar pregnancies. First-trimester diagnosis may significantly reduce the morbidity associated with these conditions by allowing for medical or minimally invasive surgical treatment which cannot be performed later in gestation.

SUMMARY

The incidence of abnormally invasive placentation resulting in placenta accreta or cesarean scar pregnancy is increasing because of the rising cesarean section rate. Women considering elective cesarean section should be counseled about the risks to future pregnancies. Obstetricians should consider the risk to future pregnancies when weighing the need for a cesarean delivery.

Placenta accreta and cesarean scar pregnancies may result in profuse hemorrhage with a risk for serious maternal morbidity and mortality, especially when this condition is not discovered until the time of delivery. A multidisciplinary approach to placenta percreta in specialized centers has the potential to improve outcomes.

Accurate diagnosis relies on a high degree of suspicion and characteristic findings on ultrasound, with MRI used when ultrasound is inconclusive or when placenta percreta is suspected. Determining the extent of placental invasion is helpful in planning the surgical approach. Early transvaginal ultrasound should be considered in patients with multiple prior cesarean sections to look for cesarean scar pregnancies. Future research may be directed at determining whether modifying surgical techniques can lower the incidence of abnormal placentation in future pregnancies.

REFERENCES

1. Hamilton BE, Martin JA, Ventura SJ. Births: preliminary data for 2006. Natl Vital Stat Rep 2007;56:1–18.

2. Smith GC, Pell JP, Cameron AD, et al. Risk of perinatal death associated with labor after previous cesarean delivery in uncomplicated term pregnancies. JAMA 2002;287:2684–90.
3. Jauniaux E, Jurkovic D, Campbell S. In vivo investigations of the anatomy and the physiology of early human placental circulations. Ultrasound Obstet Gynecol 1991;1:435–45.
4. Norwitz ER. Defective implantation and placentation: laying the blueprint for pregnancy complications. Reprod Biomed Online 2006;13:591–9.
5. Red-Horse K, Zhou Y, Genbacev O, et al. Trophoblast differentiation during embryo implantation and formation of the maternal-fetal interface. J Clin Invest 2004;114:744–54.
6. Zhou Y, Fisher SJ, Janatpour M, et al. Human cytotrophoblasts adopt a vascular phenotype as they differentiate: a strategy for successful endovascular invasion? J Clin Invest 1997;99:2139–51.
7. Genbacev O, Zhou Y, Ludlow JW, et al. Regulation of human placental development by oxygen tension. Science 1997;277:1669–72.
8. Silver RM, Landon MB, Rouse DJ, et al. Maternal morbidity associated with multiple repeat cesarean deliveries. Obstet Gynecol 2006;107:1226–32.
9. Breen JL, Neubecker R, Gregori CA, et al. Placenta accreta, increta, and percreta: a survey of 40 cases. Obstet Gynecol 1977;49:43–7.
10. Miller DA, Chollet JA, Goodwin TM. Clinical risk factors for placenta previa-placenta accreta. Am J Obstet Gynecol 1997;177:210–4.
11. Wu S, Kocherginsky M, Hibbard JU. Abnormal placentation: twenty-year analysis. Am J Obstet Gynecol 2005;192:1458–61.
12. Hoffman MK, Sciscione AC. Placenta accreta and intrauterine fetal death in a woman with prior endometrial ablation: a case report. J Reprod Med 2004; 49:384–6.
13. Pron G, Mocarski E, Bennett J, et al. Pregnancy after uterine artery embolization for leiomyomata: the Ontario multicenter trial. Obstet Gynecol 2005;105:67–76.
14. Clark SL. Placenta previa and abruptio placentae. In: Creasy RK, Resnick R, editors. Maternal-fetal medicine principles and practice. Philadelphia: Saunders; 2004. p. 616–31.
15. Zimmer EZ, Bardin R, Tamir A, et al. Sonographic imaging of cervical scars after cesarean section. Ultrasound Obstet Gynecol 2004;23:594–8.
16. Warshak CR, Eskander R, Hull AD, et al. Accuracy of ultrasonography and magnetic resonance imaging in the diagnosis of placenta accreta. Obstet Gynecol 2006;108:573–81.
17. Levine D, Hulka CA, Ludmir J, et al. Placenta accreta: evaluation with color Doppler US, power Doppler US, and MR imaging. Radiology 1997;205:773–6.
18. Chou MM, Ho ES, Lee YH. Prenatal diagnosis of placenta previa accreta by transabdominal color Doppler ultrasound. Ultrasound Obstet Gynecol 2000;15:28–35.
19. Comstock CH, Lee W, Vettraino IM, et al. The early sonographic appearance of placenta accreta. J Ultrasound Med 2003;22:19–23 [quiz 24–6].
20. Comstock CH. Antenatal diagnosis of placenta accreta: a review. Ultrasound Obstet Gynecol 2005;26:89–96.
21. Ophir E, Tendler R, Odeh M, et al. Creatine kinase as a biochemical marker in diagnosis of placenta increta and percreta. Am J Obstet Gynecol 1999;180:1039–40.
22. Hung TH, Shau WY, Hsieh CC, et al. Risk factors for placenta accreta. Obstet Gynecol 1999;93:545–50.

23. Mazouni C, Gorincour G, Juhan V, et al. Placenta accreta: a review of current advances in prenatal diagnosis. Placenta 2007;28:599–603.
24. O'Brien JM, Barton JR, Donaldson ES. The management of placenta percreta: conservative and operative strategies. Am J Obstet Gynecol 1996;175:1632–8.
25. Alfirevic Z, Elbourne D, Pavord S, et al. Use of recombinant activated factor VII in primary postpartum hemorrhage: the Northern European registry 2000–2004. Obstet Gynecol 2007;110:1270–8.
26. Dildy GA, Scott JR, Saffer CS, et al. An effective pressure pack for severe pelvic hemorrhage. Obstet Gynecol 2006;108:1222–6.
27. Timmermans S, van Hof AC, Duvekot JJ. Conservative management of abnormally invasive placentation. Obstet Gynecol Surv 2007;62:529–39.
28. Larsen JV, Solomon MH. Pregnancy in a uterine scar sacculus—an unusual cause of postabortal haemorrhage. A case report. S Afr Med J 1978;53:142–3.
29. Ash A, Smith A, Maxwell D. Caesarean scar pregnancy. BJOG 2007;114:253–63.
30. Jurkovic D, Hillaby K, Woolfer B, et al. First-trimester diagnosis and management of pregnancies implanted into the lower uterine segment cesarean section scar. Ultrasound Obstet Gynecol 2003;21:220–7.
31. Seow KM, Huang LW, Lin YH, et al. Cesarean scar pregnancy: issues in management. Ultrasound Obstet Gynecol 2004;23:247–53.
32. Fylstra DL. Ectopic pregnancy within a cesarean scar: a review. Obstet Gynecol Surv 2002;57:537–43.
33. Herman A, Weinraub Z, Avrech O, et al. Follow up and outcome of isthmic pregnancy located in a previous caesarean section scar. Br J Obstet Gynaecol 1995;102:839–41.
34. Smith L, Mueller P. Abdominal pain and hemoperitoneum in the gravid patient: a case report of placenta percreta. Am J Emerg Med 1996;14:45–7.
35. Liang HS, Jeng CJ, Sheen TC, et al. First-trimester uterine rupture from a placenta percreta: a case report. J Reprod Med 2003;48:474–0.
36. Godin PA, Bassil S, Donnez J. An ectopic pregnancy developing in a previous caesarean section scar. Fertil Steril 1997;67:398–400.
37. Hwu YM, Hsu CY, Yang HY. Conservative treatment of caesarean scar pregnancy with transvaginal needle aspiration of the embryo. BJOG 2005;112:841–2.
38. Shufaro Y, Nadjari M. Implantation of a gestational sac in a cesarean section scar. Fertil Steril 2001;75:1217.
39. Wang CJ, Yuen LT, Chao AS, et al. Caesarean scar pregnancy successfully treated by operative hysteroscopy and suction curettage. BJOG 2005;112:839–40.
40. Wang YL, Su TH, Chen HS. Operative laparoscopy for unruptured ectopic pregnancy in a caesarean scar. BJOG 2006;113:1035–8.

Mechanisms of Hemostasis at Cesarean Delivery

Clarissa Bonanno, MD*, Sreedhar Gaddipati, MD

KEYWORDS

- Hemostasis • Hemorrhage • Cesarean delivery • Uterine atony
- Medical therapy • Uterotonic agents • Surgical therapy

Postpartum hemorrhage constitutes a major cause of maternal morbidity and mortality worldwide. Annually, obstetric hemorrhage causes an estimated 140,000 maternal deaths.[1–3] Most of these deaths occur in Africa and Asia, primarily as a result of postpartum hemorrhage.[1,2] Decreasing maternal mortality is an important and continued focus of international public health efforts. In the last century, maternal deaths from hemorrhage in the developed world have decreased significantly. The introductions of blood product replacement, improved surgical techniques, and advances in critical care medicine have contributed to this welcome decline. Hemorrhage remains the second most common cause of pregnancy-related mortality in the United States, however, and accounts for approximately 17% of all maternal deaths.[4]

Prompt recognition and proper management of hemorrhage at the time of cesarean delivery are becoming increasingly more important for providers of obstetrics. In the last decade alone, the cesarean delivery rate has increased more than 50% in the United States—from 20.7% in 1996 to 31.1% in 2006.[5,6] Many factors have been implicated in this rise, including obstetric factors (eg, the decline in vaginal birth after cesarean delivery and operative vaginal delivery), maternal factors (eg, the increasing rates of obesity and mothers of advanced maternal age), and medicolegal concerns. Similar trends have been seen in many other areas of the world, from the United Kingdom to China.[7,8]

This article focuses on the etiology, risk factors, and management of hemorrhage at the time of cesarean delivery. Medical and surgical interventions can improve maternal outcomes of obstetric hemorrhage after cesarean delivery.

DEFINITION

There is no precise definition for postpartum hemorrhage. The lack of a standardized method of defining and measuring obstetric hemorrhage affects clinical practice and

---

Division of Maternal Fetal Medicine, Columbia Presbyterian Medical Center, 622 West 168th Street, PH-16, New York, NY 10032, USA
* Corresponding author.
E-mail address: cab90@columbia.edu (C. Bonanno).

Clin Perinatol 35 (2008) 531–547
doi:10.1016/j.clp.2008.07.007
perinatology.theclinics.com
0095-5108/08/$ – see front matter © 2008 Elsevier Inc. All rights reserved.

hinders research efforts into this condition. The average blood loss after cesarean delivery has been shown to be 1000 mL.[9] Traditionally, postpartum hemorrhage after cesarean delivery has been defined as any loss more than this amount. Clinical estimation of blood loss at delivery is notoriously inaccurate, however. Visual estimation has been shown to be inexact; this assessment is further complicated by the presence of amniotic fluid.[10,11] Estimates of blood loss are usually underestimated, with greater discrepancies occurring as blood loss increases.

A decline in hematocrit level of 10% after delivery has been proposed as a definition of postpartum hemorrhage.[12] Although potentially useful for quality assurance and research, this retrospective laboratory diagnosis is not valuable in the acute management of obstetric hemorrhage. Hemoconcentration resulting from intrapartum dehydration or pre-eclampsia also may lead to a significant fall in hematocrit in the postpartum period in the absence of significant blood loss. In addition, this degree of decline may not lead to symptoms in all patients.

Severe hemorrhage can also be defined by the requirement of blood transfusion or excessive bleeding that results in symptoms (dizziness, syncope) or signs (hypotension, tachycardia, oliguria) of hypovolemia. Both of these definitions are influenced by a patient's overall health and preoperative status, but they represent the best descriptions available. In most cases, the degree of hemodynamic compromise or shock parallels the volume of blood lost. Most women experience only mild symptoms with no signs of hypovolemia after blood loss of 1000 mL (15% of blood volume). Conversely, a loss of 3000 mL (45% of blood volume) leads to severe shock and cardiovascular collapse in most patients, however.

FREQUENCY OF HEMORRHAGE

The incidence of postpartum hemorrhage varies greatly and depends on the criteria used to define this condition. Primary postpartum hemorrhage, hemorrhage within the first 24 hours after delivery, occurs after approximately 4% to 6% of all deliveries.[12] Excessive bleeding after this time is referred to as secondary postpartum hemorrhage. Primary postpartum hemorrhage is generally associated with more significant bleeding and greater morbidity and is the focus of this article.

In the large prospective cohort study on cesarean delivery by the Maternal Fetal Medicine Units Network, 2.6% of approximately 57,000 women studied received a transfusion.[13] More women received a blood transfusion after primary cesarean delivery (3.2%) than repeat cesarean delivery (2.2%), probably because women who undergo a primary cesarean delivery have other risk factors for hemorrhage, including the presence of labor. These relatively low cesarean-associated transfusion rates are similar to previous studies.

IMPACT OF PREGNANCY ON HEMOSTASIS

Several physiologic changes occur over the course of pregnancy in anticipation of blood loss at delivery. Maternal blood volume expands by 40% to 50% during pregnancy as the result of increases in plasma volume and red cell mass. Fibrinogen increases markedly, as do several other procoagulant factors, which leads to the hypercoagulable state of pregnancy. These changes protect the mother from consequences of blood loss and facilitate hemostasis postpartum.[9]

Blood flow to the gravid uterus at term is approximately 800 to 1000 mL/min. Without an efficient mechanism of decreasing this flow, the previously mentioned adaptations would be insufficient to prevent maternal exsanguination. Control of postpartum bleeding occurs primarily through contraction of the myometrium surrounding the spiral arteries of the placental bed. Contraction of these interlacing myometrial fibers leads to compression of the spiral arteries and veins, obliteration of vessel lumina, and reduction of blood flow. In conjunction with systemic coagulation factors, local decidual hemostatic factors, such as tissue factor and type 1 plasminogen activator inhibitor, contribute to hemostasis.[14,15]

CAUSES OF HEMORRHAGE AT CESAREAN DELIVERY
Uterine Atony

The most common cause of postpartum hemorrhage—contributing to more than 80% of cases—is uterine atony.[16] Uterine atony refers to poor tone of the uterine musculature, which results in continued blood flow from the vasculature supplying the placental bed. There are many risk factors for uterine atony. Uterine overdistention caused by multiple gestation, macrosomia, or polyhydramnios can lead to atony, as can the use of uterine relaxants, such as general anesthetic agents and tocolytics. In the Maternal Fetal Medicine Units study on cesarean delivery and transfusion, exposure to general anesthesia increased the odds of transfusion four- to sevenfold.[13] Prolonged labor, oxytocin use, and chorioamnionitis have been associated with uterine atony.[17,18] The presence of large fibroids may interfere with the ability of the myometrium to contract. Finally, a history of postpartum hemorrhage increases the risk of hemorrhage in a subsequent pregnancy approximately threefold.[16]

Uterine atony can affect a focal area of the uterus. The lower uterine segment and cervix have a paucity of myometrial fibers. Because control of bleeding after delivery occurs primarily through myometrial contraction, spiral arteries in the lower segment cannot be compressed as effectively. In addition, as medical treatment of uterine atony is mainly targeted at enhancing myometrial contraction, the lower segment may not respond appropriately to this therapy.

Placenta Accreta

Placenta accreta is another cause of postpartum hemorrhage and is discussed in detail in Rosen's article elsewhere in this issue. The incidence of placenta accreta is increasing, representing approximately 1 in 2500 deliveries.[19] This increase can be attributed mainly to the rising cesarean delivery rate. The degree and rapid nature of blood loss in cases of placenta accreta can be massive.

Trauma

Trauma-related bleeding usually occurs secondary to uterine rupture or lacerations at the time of cesarean delivery. Lower uterine segment extensions may occur because of deep engagement of the fetal head into the pelvis, which leads to tearing at the time of delivery. As cesarean delivery continues to replace operative vaginal delivery for the management of second-stage arrest, this complication will likely occur more frequently. Operative or traumatic injury to adjacent vascular structures, such as the uterine artery or broad ligament vessels, can contribute to hemorrhage. The main risk factor for uterine rupture is previous uterine surgery, primarily cesarean delivery. A trial of labor in an attempt to accomplish a vaginal birth after a cesarean delivery increases this risk.[20]

Coagulation Abnormalities

Abnormalities in the maternal coagulation mechanism can contribute to postpartum hemorrhage. Patients who have pre-existing coagulation disorders, such as von Willebrand's disease, idiopathic thrombocytopenia purpura, and specific factor deficiencies, are at increased risk for bleeding. These patients should be evaluated early in pregnancy to develop a management plan for pregnancy, delivery, and the postpartum period. Disseminated intravascular coagulation can develop suddenly and unexpectedly and can lead to severe postpartum hemorrhage. Initiating factors for disseminated intravascular coagulation include placental abruption, amniotic fluid embolism, sepsis, and prolonged fetal demise. Patients who develop HELLP syndrome (hemolytic, elevated liver enzymes, low platelets) are at an increased risk of hemorrhage because of thrombocytopenia. Women who receive anticoagulation treatment during pregnancy also have an increased risk of hemorrhage. In most cases, a plan to discontinue or modify these medications before delivery minimizes this risk. Occasionally, an unanticipated complication, such as abruption or preterm delivery, precludes appropriate adjustment of these medications appropriately. More infrequently, a medical complication of pregnancy, such as recent venous thromboembolism or presence of mechanical heart valves, requires that anticoagulation therapy be continued through delivery.[21]

MANAGEMENT OF HEMORRHAGE AT THE TIME OF CESAREAN DELIVERY
General Principles for the Management of Cesarean Hemorrhage

Fortunately, many women with risk factors have uncomplicated cesarean deliveries and do not experience postpartum hemorrhage. Conversely, the presence of risk factors does not identify all women who hemorrhage at the time of cesarean delivery, which implies that management protocols and adequate resources must be place at all times. Drills to practice the management of obstetric hemorrhage have been shown to increase the preparedness of the team and decrease patient morbidity.[22] For patients at the highest risk for hemorrhage, such as women with the antenatal diagnosis of placenta accreta, extensive preoperative planning should be implemented.

When hemorrhage occurs, the first step should be to call for help from additional obstetric providers and nursing and anesthesia staff members. Other consultants, such as gynecologic oncologists and interventional radiologists, should be notified and attend as needed. Uterotonic agents and additional surgical instruments should be made available immediately. A rapid infuser for blood transfusion or a cell-saver device may prove helpful. The blood bank should be contacted to request blood products urgently. We have found that developing an "obstetric hemorrhage" code with the blood bank—similar to that used for trauma cases—improves the rapid availability of blood and ensures that these cases receive immediate attention.

Resuscitation of the patient should begin by obtaining adequate large bore intravenous access. Crystalloid solution is administered for volume maintenance before blood transfusion. Oxygen should be administered by face mask, and vital signs should be observed continuously. A Foley catheter should be placed if not already present. Depending on the patient's status, conversion to general anesthesia may be necessary. Laboratory tests, including complete blood count, coagulation studies, and fibrinogen level, should be performed. In many situations, however, the length of time required to perform these tests limits their usefulness in acute hemorrhage; a response to the bleeding is usually required before results are known. Bedside testing of the coagulation status may be useful. To accomplish this, a venous sample of the patient's blood is drawn into a red top tube. If 5 mL does not clot within 10 minutes, the patient's fibrinogen is less than 150 mg/dL.[23]

Concurrent with these interventions, the cause of hemorrhage should be assessed. At the time of cesarean delivery, the primary reason for hemorrhage is uterine atony, but other sources should be sought. In most cases, the diagnosis of placenta accreta or genital tract lacerations is obvious, but a search for retained products or occult lacerations may be required. The management of hemorrhage then depends on the primary cause.

Medical Therapy for Hemorrhage

Uterotonic agents

Several medications are currently available for treatment of uterine atony, including oxytocin (Pitocin), methylergonovine maleate (Methergine), carboprost tromethamine (15 methyl prostaglandin $F_{2\alpha}$, Hemabate), and misoprostol (Cytotec). With proper use of medical therapy for postpartum atony, surgical therapy often can be avoided. Despite the apparent effectiveness of these medications in the treatment of postpartum atony, evidence of their efficacy from randomized controlled trials is limited. These medications came into active clinical use before they were rigorously studied for postpartum atony and hemorrhage, which makes further critical assessment more difficult.

Pitocin is a synthetic hormone identical to the oxytocin secreted by the posterior pituitary. Oxytocin causes the upper segment of the uterus to contract in a rhythmic fashion. As more oxytocin receptors are expressed over the course of gestation, the effect of exogenous oxytocin increases. Oxytocin is typically administered after delivery of the infant at the time of cesarean delivery for prevention of postpartum hemorrhage.

Because of its short plasma half-life (mean 3 minutes), a continuous infusion of oxytocin is necessary to maintain uterine contraction. The standard protocol calls for an intravenous infusion of 10 to 40 U in 1 L of normal saline or Ringer's lactate, with the dosage rate adjusted to the uterine response (average 125–50 mL/h). Oxytocin may be injected intramuscularly in a dose of 10 U, which results in a slower onset of action (3–7 minutes) but a longer clinical effect (up to 60 minutes). The optimal dose and infusion rate have not been determined, despite widespread use of oxytocin after delivery. Increased doses of oxytocin are often given for postpartum atony and hemorrhage, despite a lack of supporting data. A recent randomized controlled trial that compared higher and lower infusion rates found that administration of high-dose oxytocin reduces the need for additional uterotonic agents but does not impact estimated blood loss, postpartum hematocrit, or transfusion rates.[24]

Rapid intravenous administration of undiluted oxytocin can result in relaxation of vascular smooth muscle, causing hypotension. Water intoxication is also a theoretic risk of the drug because of its antidiuretic effect. Side effects are rare, however, and there are no contraindications to use of oxytocin for treatment of postpartum atony.

Methylergonovine maleate (Methergine) is an ergot alkaloid that produces sustained contraction of the uterus via stimulation of myometrial α-adrenergic receptors. Methylergonovine is administered intramuscularly in a dose of 0.2 mg. It promotes contraction of the upper and lower segments of the uterus and has an onset of action of approximately 2 to 5 minutes. Although some authors advocate administration of methylergonovine every 5 minutes to a maximum of 1 mg, this dosage regimen has not been well studied.[25] The American College of Obstetrics and Gynecology[12] cites a dosage regimen of 0.2 mg every 2 to 4 hours in its practice bulletin on postpartum hemorrhage. Methylergonovine may also be administered into the uterus at the time of cesarean delivery. Side effects include nausea and vomiting. Methylergonovine may cause peripheral vasoconstriction and is contraindicated in patients with chronic hypertension or hypertensive disorders of pregnancy.

Carboprost tromethamine (Hemabate) is a synthetic 15 methyl analog of prostaglandin $F_{2\alpha}$, which acts as a smooth muscle stimulant. Carboprost is administered as an intramuscular or intramyometrial injection in doses of 0.25 mg. These injections can be repeated every 15 minutes to a maximum of 2 mg (eight doses). Peak plasma concentrations are obtained at 5 minutes through the intramyometrial route versus 15 minutes via peripheral muscular injection. It is an effective agent for increasing uterine tone; several case series have demonstrated success rates of 84% to 96% using carboprost for refractory postpartum hemorrhage.[25] Prostaglandin side effects are frequent, however, and include nausea, vomiting, diarrhea, fever, and hypertension. Life-threatening bronchospasm has occurred after carboprost administration, and use of this medication is contraindicated in patients with asthma. Relative contraindications include cardiac, renal, and hepatic disease.

Misoprostol is a synthetic analog of prostaglandin E_1. There are multiple routes of administration for misoprostol: oral, sublingual, vaginal, and rectal. Misoprostol should not be administered vaginally for postpartum hemorrhage, because bleeding is likely to limit absorption of the drug. Rectal misoprostol has a more favorable side-effect profile than the oral or sublingual route. Although rectal misoprostol has a longer onset of action than oral or sublingual misoprostol, this route of administration is most practical for women with acute hemorrhage. The typical dose of rectal misoprostol is 800 to 1000 μg.

Three randomized controlled trials for treatment of primary postpartum hemorrhage were cited by a Cochrane review, all of which involved misprostol.[26] Two of these studies compared misoprostol with placebo when bleeding persisted despite the use of conventional uterotonics, and the other compared misoprostol to combined oxytocics (Syntometrine [5 U oxytocin and 0.5 mg *ergometrine maleate*] and oxytocin infusion) for primary postpartum hemorrhage. The number of women in these studies was too small to evaluate the effect of treatment with misoprostol on maternal mortality, serious morbidity, or need for hysterectomy. Misoprostol use was associated with a significant reduction in blood loss of 500 mL or more, although there were no differences in any other outcomes assessed. The authors concluded that additional, larger studies are necessary to determine the efficacy of these agents for postpartum hemorrhage.

There are many advantages to misoprostol with respect to cost, stability, and ease of administration. Neither intravenous access nor sterile needles are required. Although these attributes make misoprostol the ideal candidate for use in the developing world, these characteristics are valuable for use in all obstetric settings. Unlike methylergonovine and carboprost, misoprostol can be administered to women with hypertension or asthma. Fever and shivering are reported side effects of misoprostol. Gastrointestinal side effects, such as nausea, vomiting, and diarrhea, can result, although less commonly after rectal administration.

Recombinant activated factor VII

Recombinant activated factor VII (rFVIIa, NovoSeven) was developed to promote hemostasis in patients with hemophilia with inhibitors to factor VIII or factor VI. rFVIIa is also approved for the prevention and treatment of bleeding in patients with congenital factor VII deficiency. As experience with this agent has grown, rFVIIa has been used increasingly "off label" for nonhemophilic bleeding conditions, including intracerebral hemorrhage, coagulopathy related to liver dysfunction, and trauma. rFVIIa has been used successfully to treat obstetric hemorrhage refractory to conventional treatment. Increasing evidence supports the efficacy and safety of this medication for obstetric hemorrhage, although the literature is still limited to case reports and case series.

The mechanism of action of rFVIIa is not completely understood. Initially rFVIIa was believed to take advantage of the normal tissue factor/FVII-dependent extrinsic coagulation pathway. In this model of hemostasis, vessel wall damage exposes tissue factor (tissue thromboplastin) to the circulating blood. Tissue factor is the cofactor required for the production of factor VIIa, and the tissue factor-FVIIa complex activates factors IX and X, which lead to the production of thrombin and fibrin. Experimental data also support a tissue factor–independent mechanism of action, however, in which rFVIIa directly activates FX on platelet surfaces in a dose-dependent fashion.[27] Understanding of these mechanisms helps to explain the therapeutic effect of rFVIIa in a range of coagulation disorders and the localization of effect to sites of bleeding.

In 2001, Moscardo and colleagues[28] published a report on the first successful use of rFVIIa for severe obstetric hemorrhage. The patient presented with disseminated intra-vascular coagulation with a twin pregnancy at 31 weeks' gestation. A cesarean delivery was performed; however, her postoperative course was complicated by intra-abdominal bleeding and worsening disseminated intravascular coagulation. Her status did not improve despite hysterectomy and massive blood product transfusion. rFVIIa was then administered at a dose of 90 μg/kg. Good clinical response was noted after the second dose, and nine total doses were administered. The patient recovered completely without experiencing any side effects of rFVIIa administration.

Ahonen and Jokela[29] reported success in 11 of 12 cases in which rFVIIa was used for severe obstetric hemorrhage. Six of 11 patients had only a partial response, however, 4 of whom required subsequent selective arterial embolization. With increasing experience using rFVIIa over the course of the study, the authors administered rFVIIa earlier in the bleeding episode. This practice resulted in decreased total blood loss and total blood products transfused over the course of the study. Franchini and colleagues[27] recently summarized the literature on rFVIIa for postpartum hemor-rhage. Their review detailed the outcomes of 118 patients from 31 studies. The primary causes of hemorrhage were uterine atony (28.0%), uterine or vaginal lacera tions (18.6%), and placental abnormalities (14.1%). Postpartum hemorrhage occurred more frequently after cesarean delivery than vaginal delivery (57.4% versus 42.6%).

rFVIIa was reported to be effective in approximately 90% of cases. In most cases a single dose of rFVIIa was given (median 1.6, range 1–19) at a median dose of 71.6 μg/kg (range 10–170 μg/kg). rFVIIa was often used after standard medical and surgical treatment, including hysterectomy; in some cases, use of the agent may have been effective in avoiding hysterectomy in some cases. Noting significant publication bias, the authors advised caution in interpreting these successful outcomes. Further evidence from randomized controlled trials is needed to clarify the optimal dose, effectiveness, and safety of rFVIIa for obstetric hemorrhage. Based on this review and their experience with the drug, the authors provided several recommendations:

- Standard medical and conservative surgical interventions should be used in the case of severe obstetric hemorrhage
- Administration of rFVIIa should be considered before proceeding with hysterectomy
- rFVIIa in a dose of 60–90 μg/kg should be given; this dose may be repeated within 30 minutes if there is a lack of clinical improvement

Extensive evidence supports the safety of rFVIIa for use in patients who have hemo-philia; however, there is a risk of arterial and venous thrombotic events related to administration of rFVIIa. Most of the thrombotic complications from use of rFVIIa have been associated with off-label use and seem to be related to a higher cumulative dose. Researchers recommend that rFVIIa be used cautiously in patients with other risk factors for thrombosis, including pregnancy.

Hemostatic agents

At the time of surgery, hemostasis can typically be achieved through a combination of pressure, electrocoagulation, and suture ligation. Topical hemostatic agents are often helpful in achieving adequate hemostasis, however, particularly for patients with an acquired or inherited coagulopathy. These products are not useful in the standard medical management of obstetric hemorrhage; however, they can be helpful in achieving adequate hemostasis after hysterectomy.

Mechanical and active hemostatic agents are available for use.[30,31] Mechanical agents allow platelet aggregation and coagulation by providing a meshwork on which clotting can take place. Most of the active agents contain thrombin alone or in combination with other procoagulant agents. Some of these agents have broad US Food and Drug Administration approval for hemostasis during surgical procedures, whereas others would be used off label in obstetric patients. The following mechanical agents are currently available:

Gelatin (Gelfoam): Purified gelatin solution is available in several different vehicles, including powders, sponges, and sheets. Gelatin provides effective hemostasis for small-vessel oozing and can be augmented with thrombin for enhanced efficacy.

Cellulose (Oxycel, Surgicel): Oxidized regenerated cellulose is produced from plant fiber and is available in different vehicles.

Collagen (Avitene): This bovine microfibrillar collagen product is available in different vehicles. Products must be kept dry and applied with pressure to the bleeding area; however, they may be more effective at achieving hemostasis than the other mechanical agents.

The following are active agents:

Thrombin (Thrombostat or Thrombin-JMI): Thrombin promotes the conversion of fibrinogen to fibrin, a key element in clot formation. Bovine thrombin is available as a solution or powder that can be applied directly to the bleeding field.

Fibrin sealants: These agents combine thrombin and fibrinogen, which act together to form fibrin. Tisseel, the first surgical sealant introduced in the United States, consists of heat-treated pooled plasma thrombin and fibrinogen. Evicel is a second-generation plasma product that is reduced in plasminogen and eliminates the need for a potentially allergenic stabilizer. Vitagel combines bovine thrombin with autologous plasma and does not contain pooled donor blood. Theoretically, Tisseel and Evicel carry the risk of viral transmission, although the products are treated with ultrafiltration, heat, and solvent detergent to decrease that risk. No cases of infection from these products have been proven.

Gelatin and thrombin (FloSeal): This product is a combination of bovine collagen and pooled human thrombin. Once applied, the bleeding area can be compressed with a surgical sponge. The product causes coagulation at the site in conjunction with pressure, but it does not stick to the sponge itself. Excess product can be washed away after hemostasis is achieved without compromising the effect.

Albumin and glutaraldehyde (BioGlue): This product is another two-component surgical adhesive that contains bovine serum albumin cross-linked with glutaraldehyde. The glutaraldehyde molecules cross-link the bovine serum albumin and tissue proteins at the repair site to create a seal independent of the coagulation process. This effective sealant is approved for the open repair of large vessels.

Surgical Therapy for Hemorrhage

When medical therapy does not prove effective, a surgical approach is required. Although hysterectomy ultimately should control postpartum hemorrhage, several other approaches attempt to manage hemorrhage while preserving fertility.

Compressive techniques

These approaches encourage the uterine myometrium to compress spiral arteries and venous sinuses that supply the placental bed. Uterine packing was the first technique used for this purpose. More recently, intrauterine balloon placement has been described to decrease uterine bleeding in a similar manner. Many different suture compressive techniques are described in the literature, with the B-Lynch suture most commonly used.

Uterine packing

Uterine packing was performed often in the earlier half of the twentieth century. The technique fell out of favor, however, because of concerns regarding infection and concealed hemorrhage. There was also concern that the process of packing interfered with the physiologic processes of uterine contraction and involution.[26] Even as the practice was falling out of favor, however, data were accumulating to support its effectiveness. In 1956, Pierce and Winkler[32] reported 505 cases of postpartum hemorrhage treated with uterine packing, with none of the cohort needing hysterectomy. In 1960, Taylor[33] credited the practice of uterine packing with preventing hysterectomy for severe atony, spanning a period of 15 years and nearly 65,000 deliveries. Later articles also lent support to the use of this practice.[34-36]

Proper technique is essential for uterine packing to be effective. The uterus should be filled from the fundus to the cervix. The packing must be tight and symmetrically placed to fill all contours of the uterine cavity, and the vagina should be packed. Should extra gauze be needed, gauze rolls may be tied to each other. The gauze may be soaked in thrombin before placement for additional effectiveness (5000 U of thrombin in 5 ml sterile saline). Placement of the packing necessitates placement of a urinary Foley catheter. Although the optimal time for packing removal is not defined, it seems reasonable to remove the pack within 24 to 36 hours, assuming the patient is hemodynamically stable. In all cases, the number of gauze pads should be counted and all pads accounted for at the time of removal. Prophylactic antibiotics may be used to decrease the rate of endometritis, although the benefit is not proven in randomized studies.

Intrauterine balloon placement

Several reports have described intrauterine compression with balloon devices to control postpartum hemorrhage.[37,38] The Sengstaken-Blakemore tube has been used successfully to treat refractory postpartum hemorrhage.[39,40] Designed for the management of esophageal variceal bleeding, the tube is modified by removing the distal tip of the tube superior to the balloon. It is then inserted into the uterine cavity and inflated. Compression of the uterine cavity and placental bed promotes hemostasis. Recently, Condous and colleagues[41] suggested that the Sengstaken-Blakemore tube be used as a "tamponade test" in the management of hemorrhage. In their series of 16 women, 14 responded to placement of the Sengstaken-Blakemore tube and did not need further surgery. The 2 patients who failed to respond required further surgical intervention.

Bakri and colleagues[42,43] designed an intrauterine balloon that promised to conform better to the contour of the uterine cavity (SOS Bakri Tamponade Balloon Catheter,

Cook Medical, Bloomington, Indiana). The Bakri balloon resembles a Foley catheter; however, it has an opening at its distal end that allows the intrauterine contents to drain. This feature may decrease the likelihood of a concealed hemorrhage within the cavity in the case of tamponade failure. The balloon is inflated with 500 mL saline, and the catheter is either secured to the leg or attached to a weight to provide traction and compression of the balloon against the lower uterine segment. Success at arresting hemorrhage has been demonstrated with intrauterine balloon placement, although no randomized studies have been performed to compare various balloon devices.

Suture techniques

In 1997, B-Lynch and colleagues[44] reported a new method of compressing the uterus. For detailed descriptions of the suture, the reader is referred to articles by the author or the Web site at www.cbl.uk.com.

In summary, the abdomen most be opened and the uterus exteriorized. A low transverse hysterotomy incision is created if not already present, and after determining that there is no retained placental tissue or blood clots, the uterus is manually compressed. If the bleeding decreases with compression, the patient is a candidate for this procedure. The B-lynch suture was initially described using No. 2 chromic catgut. In later reports, poliglecaprone 25 monofilament (Monocryl) was used. The suture is made by entering the anterior uterine wall 3 cm below the hysterotomy and exiting 3 cm above the incision. The suture is then looped over the fundus and brought in and out of the posterior uterine wall at the level of the uterosacral ligaments. The suture is again brought over the fundus on the opposite side of the uterus, giving the appearance of suspenders. Finally, the suture is passed 3 cm above the hysterotomy and exits 3 cm below. With continued manual compression the suture is tied.

Since the initial publication of this suture technique, approximately 1800 cases have been reported with few failures.[45,46] Two cases of uterine necrosis that required hysterectomy after B-lynch suture placement were reported.[47,48] Whether these adverse outcomes resulted from improper technique has been debated.[47,49,50] The overwhelming success of the B-lynch suture may be related to publication bias and underreporting of suture failures, but there is no doubt that this is a valuable procedure in the management of severe atony. Several authors have described modifications of the B-lynch technique.[51,52] Hayman and colleagues[51] described placement of two to four vertical compression sutures without hysterotomy. A separate cervicoisthmic suture may be placed to control bleeding from the lower uterine segment if necessary. Nelson and Birch[52] also reported on a modification of the B-Lynch suture in which the needle is passed through the uterine fundus to prevent the sutures from slipping off laterally.

Cho and colleagues[53] described a hemostatic square suture technique, which is performed by passing the suture through the uterus, entering the anterior uterine wall, and exiting the posterior uterine wall. The needle is then brought back and forth through the uterus to form a 2- to 3-cm square that is tied interiorly. Multiple square sutures can be placed to compress the corpus of the uterus. The authors described use of this suture for uterine atony in 23 women. After a short period of follow-up, these women were noted to have normal endometrial stripes by ultrasound, normal uterine cavities by uterine sounding, and resumption of normal menstrual flow. Six of ten women who desired future pregnancy had a hysterosalpingogram or hysteroscopy that documented normal cavities. Subsequently, four of these women had successful pregnancies. Pyometria was reported 4 weeks postpartum in a patient whose delivery was also complicated by endometritis.[54] A curettage was performed for evacuation of purulent material, and a hysterosalpingogram performed 5 months postpartum revealed Asherman's syndrome. Wu and Yeh[55] also noted a case of Asherman's syndrome that may have been related to the polyglycolic acid suture (Dexon) used with the Cho technique.

Hackethal and colleagues[56] reported on successful use of horizontal U sutures. In seven patients, polyglactin (Vicryl) was passed from the anterior uterine wall through the posterior uterine wall and back, with the knot tied anteriorly. Hwu and colleagues[57] reported on the use of vertical U sutures in the lower uterine segment of patients. In this description, the suture was only passed superficially into the posterior uterine wall and was effective in controlling bleeding in patients with placenta previa.

Although several of the reports commented on future pregnancies,[53,55] Baskett[58] recently reported the largest series of pregnancies after use of surgical compression techniques. Of the 28 cases at his institution, 20 women retained their uterus, and 7 had uneventful subsequent pregnancies. In 4 of these patients there appeared to be evidence of the previous surgery–either grooving of the fundus or puckering where suture entry had occurred.

In summary, these suture compression techniques have been effective in the management of postpartum hemorrhage and atony. Although B-Lynch reported that his technique has a 99% success rate, Baskett's[58] review of the literature suggests a somewhat lower success rate at avoiding hysterectomy of 86%. Most of these procedures have been performed without complication, and although future fertility seems to be preserved, it should continue to be an area of investigation.

Vessel occlusion: uterine artery and hypogastric artery ligation

Uterine artery ligation was first described in the 1950s. Waters reported that this safe and rapid procedure led to 90% reduction in blood flow and was helpful in controlling postpartum hemorrhage.[59] Although earlier authors advocated isolating the uterine arteries, O'Leary[60] reported success with mass ligation of the uterine artery and veins. The technique described uses 1-0 chromic suture placed below the level of a transverse uterine incision. The needle is passed 2 to 3 cm medial to the uterine vessels and then brought forward through an avascular portion of the broad ligament. It is then tied to compress those vessels. Ideally, the ureters are identified bilaterally before placement of the stitch.

According to a recent review of 265 cases, the technique was successful in controlling hemorrhage in more than 95% of patients.[61] The uterine arteries also may be ligated more superiorly, at the level of the utero-ovarian ligament, to decrease bleeding from ovarian artery anastomoses. AbdRabbo[62] reported on stepwise uterine vessel ligation, with the steps including: unilateral uterine vessel ligation → bilateral uterine vessel ligation → low bilateral uterine vessel ligation → unilateral ovarian vessel ligation → bilateral ovarian vessel ligation. Of 102 women managed with this technique, no hysterectomies were performed and no complications were noted. In 75% of cases, hemorrhage was controlled with bilateral uterine vessel ligation. Only 6% of cases required bilateral ovarian vessel ligation. No cases of subsequent ovarian failure developed in these patients.

Acute complications from uterine artery ligation can occur and include broad ligament hematoma. Injury to the ureter is also possible, particularly with low uterine vessel ligation. Because the suture used is not permanent, recanalization of the vessels is expected, without compromise of fertility. No cases of uterine necrosis or fetal growth restriction in subsequent pregnancies have been reported. Case reports have noted intrauterine synechiae and ovarian failure after ligation, however, including the ovarian vessels.[63,64]

Hypogastric artery ligation for postpartum hemorrhage was first reported in the 1950s. Burchell's[65] seminal work published in 1964 elucidated the hemodynamics of the internal iliac artery. Burchell showed that pulse pressure decreased approximately 85% after bilateral hypogastric artery ligation. With unilateral ligation, the pulse pressure decreased 77% on the same side but only 14% on the opposite side. The dramatic effect from bilateral ligation was described as "a transformation of the pelvic circulation into a sluggish venous-like system." Despite the dramatic reduction in blood flow, the success of hypogastric artery ligation is limited. The success rates in reducing hemorrhage and preventing hysterectomy are between 43% and 67%.[66–69] In a recent report, Joshi and colleagues[69] reviewed the outcomes of 110 women who underwent hypogastric artery ligation, with 66.8% avoiding hysterectomy or repeat laparotomy. Use of hypogastric artery ligation did not effectively reduce hemorrhage caused by uterine rupture (22% success rate) or atony after vaginal delivery (43% success rate). Hypogastric artery ligation was most effective for atony after cesarean delivery (85%). Subsequent ligation of the utero-ovarian ligament may also improve success rates.[70]

This technique requires a knowledge of the vascular, ureteral, and neuroanatomy of the pelvis. The technique is difficult, especially in the circumstances of a Pfannensteil incision, an enlarged uterus, and significant blood in the pelvis. Currently many obstetric providers do not have adequate training in this procedure, particularly for performance in an emergent situation. Uterine artery ligation has largely replaced this procedure because of the technical ease and improved success rate. Hypogastric artery ligation should be performed only after other medical and surgical interventions have failed, and this procedure should not significantly delay hysterectomy. Consultation with a gynecologic oncologist, who routinely operates in the retroperitoneum, may be considered.

Technically, the retroperitoneum is entered by opening the broad ligament. The external iliac artery is found medial to the psoas muscle and is followed to the iliac bifurcation. The ureter is expected to cross over the vessels at the iliac bifurcation, and when identified, it is mobilized medially. The internal iliac artery is identified and ligated approximately 2 cm distal to the origin. A free ligature of 0 silk is passed lateral to medial (to avoid the internal iliac vein) and tied. The anterior division is selectively ligated when possible, although the challenges listed previously make this procedure difficult. There are several serious risks of this procedure, including ischemia of the gluteal muscles (from ligation of the posterior division), injury to the ureter, accidental ligation of the external iliac artery leading to ischemia of the lower limb, and laceration of the internal iliac vein.[66,69] Fertility does not seem to be compromised after hypogastric artery ligation.[71]

Selective arterial embolization/balloon occlusion

The use of interventional radiology to localize and occlude bleeding vessels has been performed since the 1960s. Use of these procedures in obstetrics was first described in 1979.[72] Several different hemostatic materials can be used. Gelfoam (gelatin) pledgets are commonly used because of ease of use, low cost, and resorption within 7 to 21 days.[73] Some authors have reported success with the addition of embolization coils to the Gelfoam, citing better results in high-flow settings.[74] It is important to note that embolization may not be possible in patients with profuse continued hemorrhage because of the time required to perform the procedure and the availability of radiologic staff. Critically ill patients may not be suitable for transfer to the radiology suite.

In their review of 67 cases of embolization, Vedantham and colleagues[75] noted a 97% success rate in controlling hemorrhage with a 6% to 7% complication rate. Similarly, Doumouchtsis and colleagues[76] noted a success rate of 90.7% in their review of nearly 200 cases. Complications from embolization can be transient, such as low-grade fever or hematoma formation at the catheter insertion site. Rarer—but more concerning—complications have been reported, including uterine necrosis, bladder necrosis, fistula formation, neurologic injury, perforation or occlusion of the external iliac artery, and small bowel injury.[76,77] Cordonnier and colleagues[78] also reported on a case of fetal growth restriction in a woman who conceived 17 months after uterine artery embolization for postpartum hemorrhage. Because of nonreassuring fetal status, the infant was delivered at 34 weeks' gestation. Pathologic examination showed ischemia of over two-thirds of the placenta. Although conclusions cannot be drawn from a single report, it seems prudent to monitor fetal growth more frequently while long-term outcomes after embolization continue to be assessed. Other successful pregnancies have been reported after embolization, although the recurrence of hemorrhage seems high.[79]

In an attempt to minimize complications from embolization, intravascular occlusive balloon catheters have been used. An initial report by Levine and colleagues[80] showed that use of balloon catheters did not decrease blood loss, transfusion requirement, or length of hospital stay. More recent reports have confirmed these findings.[81] A recent study by Shrivastava and colleagues[82] summarized the outcomes of 69 patients with placenta accreta, 19 of whom underwent prophylactic balloon catheters placement. Catheter use did not decrease blood loss, blood product administration, or overall morbidity. Unfortunately, vessel ligation and embolization procedures may be limited in their effectiveness because of the extensive collateral blood supply to the gravid uterus. This is a particular problem in cases of placenta accreta, in which neovascularization can be extensive.

For cases of severe, life-threatening hemorrhage, a balloon catheter for aortic occlusion may be useful for decreasing blood loss and facilitating surgical correction. Although not reported in the obstetric literature, this technique has been used in other fields, notably in cases of trauma, and recently for massive hemorrhage after hepato-pancreatobiliary surgery. Because there is a risk for renal or spinal ischemia, Miura and colleagues[83] used intermittent occlusion, which did not result in any complications. Aortic compression and cross-clamping are also possible in cases of massive, life-threatening hemorrhage. The literature on these techniques for postpartum hemorrhage is limited, but we have used these techniques successfully in our center.

Hysterectomy

Hysterectomy must always be considered for definitive treatment of postpartum hemorrhage. Although this procedure is frequently considered a last resort, particularly for women who have not completed their childbearing, it may be life-saving and must be performed when other approaches do not rapidly resolve the bleeding. Patient outcomes are often worse when hysterectomy is delayed by prolonged attempts at controlling hemorrhage with medical therapy or conservative surgical techniques, because massive blood loss, even in the presence of optimal blood product replacement, can quickly lead to consumptive coagulopathy. Coagulopathy complicates the hysterectomy, with the bleeding becoming intractable to any surgical correction. In cases of profuse bleeding, rapid sequential clamping and cutting of the vascular pedicles through the level of the uterine arteries should be considered to achieve hemostasis. After the major blood supply to the uterus is controlled, the surgeon may return to perform suture ligation all of the pedicles.

SUMMARY

Postpartum hemorrhage represents an obstetric emergency. Prompt recognition and proper management at the time of cesarean delivery are becoming increasingly important for providers of obstetric care. Preparedness for hemorrhage can be achieved by recognizing prior risk factors and implementing specific protocols. A delay in diagnosis and treatment may lead to greater blood loss and greater morbidity from this condition. Medical and surgical therapies are available for the treatment of hemorrhage after cesarean delivery; however, untoward delay should not occur before proceeding to hysterectomy, because it may be a life-saving procedure.

REFERENCES

1. AbouZahr C. Global burden of maternal death and disability. Br Med Bull 2003; 67:1–11.
2. World Health Organization (WHO) Department of Reproductive Health and Research. Maternal mortality in 2005: estimates developed by WHO, UNICEF, and UNFPA. Geneva (Switzerland): WHO; 2005.
3. Khan KS, Wojdyla D, Say L, et al. WHO analysis of causes of maternal death: a systematic review. Lancet 2006;367:1066–74.
4. Kung HC, Hoyert DL, Xu J, et al. Deaths: final data for 2005. National Vital Statistics Reports 2008;56(10):1–121.
5. Menacker F, Curtin SC. Trends in cesarean and vaginal birth after previous cesarean 1991–99. National Vital Statistics Reports 2001;49(13):1–16.
6. Hamilton BE, Martin JA, Ventura SJ. Births: preliminary data for 2006. National Vital Statistics Reports 2007;56(7):1–16.
7. Black C, Kaye JA, Jick H. Cesarean delivery in the United Kingdom: time trends in the practice research database. Obstet Gynecol 2005;106:151–5.
8. Sufang G, Padmadas SS, Fengmin Z, et al. Delivery settings and cesarean section rates in China. Bull World Health Organ 2007;85:755–62.
9. Pritchard JA, Baldwin RM, Dickey JC, et al. Blood volume changes in pregnancy and the puerperium. Am J Obstet Gynecol 1962;84:1271–82.
10. Jansen AJ, Rhenen DJ, Steegers EA, et al. Postpartum hemorrhage and transfusion of blood and blood components. Obstet Gynecol Surv 2005;60:663–71.
11. Andolina K, Daly S, Roberts N, et al. Objective measurement of blood loss at delivery: is it more than a guess? Am J Obstet Gynecol 1999;180:S69.
12. American College of Obstetrics and Gynecology (ACOG) Practice Bulletin. Postpartum hemorrhage. Obstet Gynecol 2006;108:1039–48.
13. Rouse DJ, MacPherson C, Landon M, et al. Blood transfusion and cesarean delivery. Obstet Gynecol 2006;108:891–7.
14. Lockwood CJ, Shatz F. A biological model for the regulation of peri-implantation hemostasis and menstruation. J Soc Gynecol Investig 1996;3:159–65.
15. Lockwood CJ. Regulation of plasminogen activator inhibitor 1 expression by interaction of epidermal growth factor with progestin during decidualization of human endometrial stromal cells. Am J Obstet Gynecol 2001;184:798–805.
16. Combs CA, Murphy EL, Laros RK. Factors associated with postpartum hemorrhage with vaginal birth. Obstet Gynecol 1991;77:69–76.
17. Rouse DJ, Leindecker S, Landon M, et al. The MFMU cesarean registry: uterine atony after primary cesarean delivery. Am J Obstet Gynecol 2005;193:1056–60.
18. Rouse DJ, Landon M, Leveno KJ, et al. The maternal-fetal medicine units cesarean registry: chorioamnionitis at term and its duration-relationship to outcome. Am J Obstet Gynecol 2004;191:211–6.
19. Miller DA, Chollet JA, Goodwin T, et al. Clinical risk factors for placenta previa/placenta accreta. Am J Obstet Gynecol 1997;177:210–4.

20. Landon MB, Spong CY, Thom E. Risk of uterine rupture with a trial of labor in women with multiple and single prior cesarean delivery. Obstet Gynecol 2006;108:12–20.
21. Krivak TC, Zorn KK. Venous thromboembolism in obstetrics and gynecology. Obstet Gynecol 2007;109:761–77.
22. Rizvi F, Mackey R, Barrett T, et al. Successful reeducation of massive postpartum hemorrhage by use of guidelines and staff education. BJOG 2004;111:495–8.
23. Poe MF. Clot observation test for clinical diagnosis of clotting defects. Anesthesiology 1959;20:825–9.
24. Munn MB, Owen J, Vincent R. Comparison of two oxytocin regimens to prevent uterine atony at cesarean delivery: a randomized controlled trial. Obstet Gynecol 2001;98:389–90.
25. Schuurmans N, MacKinnon C, Lane C, et al. Prevention and management of postpartum hemorrhage. Journal of the Society of Obstetricians and Gynaecologists of Canada 2000;88:1–11.
26. Mousa HA, Alfirevic Z. Treatment for primary postpartum hemorrhage. Cochrane Database Syst Rev 2006;1:CD003249.
27. Franchini M, Lippi G, Franchi M. The use of recombinant activated factor VII in obstetric and gynaecological hemorrhage. BJOG 2007;114:8–15.
28. Moscardo F, Perez F, de la Rubia J, et al. Successful treatment of severe intra-abdominal bleeding associated with disseminated intravascular coagulation using recombinant activated factor VII. Br J Haematol 2001;114:174–6.
29. Ahonen J, Jokela R. Recombinant factor VIIa for life-threatening post-partum haemorrhage. Br J Anaesth 2005;94:592–5.
30. Palm MD, Altman JS. Topical hemostatic agents: a review. Dermatol Surg 2008; 34:431–45.
31. Spotnitz WD. Active and mechanical hemostatic agents. Surgery 2007;142:S34–8.
32. Pierce JR, Winkler EG. Why not pack the postpartum uterus? Minn Med 1956;39: 84–125.
33. Taylor ES. Intrapartum and postpartum hemorrhage. Clin Obstet Gynecol 1960;3: 646–65.
34. Hester JD. Postpartum hemorrhage and reevaluation of uterine packing. Obstet Gynecol 1975;45.501–4
35. Druzin ML. Packing of lower uterine segment for control of post-cesarean bleeding in instances of placenta previa. Surg Gynecol Obstet 1989;169:543–5.
36. Maier RC. Control of postpartum hemorrhage with uterine packing. Am J Obstet Gynecol 1993;169:317–21.
37. Bowen LW, Beeson JH. Use of a large Foley catheter balloon to control postpartum hemorrhage resulting from a low placental implantation: a report of two cases. J Reprod Med 1985;30:623–5.
38. Bakri YN. Uterine tamponade-drain for hemorrhage secondary to placenta previa-accreta. Int J Gynaecol Obstet 1992;37:302–3.
39. Katesmart M, Brown R, Raju KS. Successful use of a Sengstaken-Blakemore tube to control massive postpartum haemorrhage. BJOG 1994;101:259–60.
40. De Loor JA, van Dam PA. Foley catheters for uncontrollable obstetric or gynecologic hemorrhage. Obstet Gynecol 1996;88:737.
41. Condous GS, Arulkumaran S, Symonds I, et al. The "Tamponade Test" in the management of postpartum hemorrhage. Obstet Gynecol 2003;101:767–72.
42. Bakri YN. Balloon device for control of obstetrical bleeding. Eur J Obstet Gynecol Reprod Biol 1999;86:S84.
43. Bakri YN, Amri A, Abdul Jabbar F, et al. Tamponade-balloon for obstetrical bleeding. Int J Gynaecol Obstet 2001;74:139–42.

44. B-Lynch C, Coker A, Lawal AH, et al. The B-Lynch surgical technique for the control of massive postpartum haemorrhage: an alternative to hysterectomy? Five cases reported. BJOG 1997;104:372–5.

45. Allam MS, B-Lynch C. The B-Lynch and other uterine compression suture techniques. Int J Gynaecol Obstet 2005;89:236–41.

46. Price N, Lynch C. Uterine necrosis following B-Lynch suture for primary postpartum haemorrhage. BJOG 2006;113:1341–2.

47. Treloar EJ, Anderson RS, Andrews HS, et al. Uterine necrosis following B-Lynch suture for primary postpartum haemorrhage. BJOG 2006;113:486–8.

48. Joshi VM, Shrivastava M. Partial ischemic necrosis of the uterus following a uterine brace compression suture. BJOG 2004;111:279–80.

49. B-Lynch C. Partial ischemic necrosis of the uterus following a uterine brace compression suture. BJOG 2005;112:126–7.

50. El-Hamamy E. Partial ischemic necrosis of the uterus following a uterine brace compression suture. BJOG 2005;112:126.

51. Hayman RG, Arulkumaran S, Steer PJ. Uterine compression sutures: surgical management of postpartum hemorrhage. Obstet Gynecol 2002;99:502–6.

52. Nelson GS, Birch C. Compression sutures for uterine atony and hemorrhage following cesarean delivery. Int J Gynaecol Obstet 2006;92:248–50.

53. Cho JH, Jun HS, Lee CN. Hemostatic suturing technique for uterine bleeding during cesarean delivery. Obstet Gynecol 2000;96:129–31.

54. Ochoa M, Allaire AD, Stitely ML. Pyometria after hemostatic square suture technique. Obstet Gynecol 2002;99:506–9.

55. Wu HH, Yeh GP. Uterine cavity synechiae after hemostatic square suturing technique. Obstet Gynecol 2005;105:1176–8.

56. Hackethal A, Brueggmann D, Oehmke F, et al. Uterine compression U-sutures in primary postpartum hemorrhage after cesarean section: fertility preservation with a simple and effective technique. Hum Reprod 2008;23:74–9.

57. Hwu YM, Chen CP, Chen HS, et al. Parallel vertical compression sutures: a technique to control bleeding from placenta praevia or accreta during caesarean section. BJOG 2005;112:1420–3.

58. Baskett TF. Uterine compression sutures for postpartum hemorrhage: efficacy, morbidity, and subsequent pregnancy. Obstet Gynecol 2007;110:68–71.

59. Waters EG. Surgical management of postpartum hemorrhage with particular reference to ligation of uterine arteries. Am J Obstet Gynecol 1952;64:1143–8.

60. O'Leary JL, O'Leary JA. Uterine artery ligation for control of postcesarean section hemorrhage. Obstet Gynecol 1974;43:849–53.

61. O'Leary JA. Uterine artery ligation in the control of postcesarean hemorrhage. J Reprod Med 1995;40:189–93.

62. AbdRabbo SA. Stepwise uterine devascularization: a novel technique for management of uncontrolled postpartum hemorrhage with preservation of the uterus. Am J Obstet Gynecol 1994;171:694–700.

63. Roman H, Sentilhes L, Cingotti M, et al. Uterine devascularization and subsequent major intrauterine synechiae and ovarian failure. Fertil Steril 2005;83:755–7.

64. Sentilhes L, Trichot C, Resch B, et al. Fertility and pregnancy outcomes following uterine devascularization for severe postpartum haemorrhage. Hum Reprod 2008;23:1087–92.

65. Burchell RC. Internal iliac artery ligation: hemodynamics. Obstet Gynecol 1964;24:737–9.

66. Clark SL, Phelan JP, Yeh SY, et al. Hypogastric artery ligation for obstetric hemorrhage. Obstet Gynecol 1985;66:353–6.

67. Evans S, McShane P. The efficacy of internal iliac artery ligation in obstetric hemorrhage. BJOG 1985;160:250–3.
68. Chattopadhyay SK, Deb Roy B, Edrees YB. Surgical control of obstetric hemorrhage: hypogastric artery ligation or hysterectomy? Int J Gynaecol Obstet 1990; 32:345–51.
69. Joshi VM, Otiv SR, Majumder R, et al. Internal iliac artery ligation for arresting postpartum haemorrhage. Br J Obstet Gynaecol 2007;114:356–61.
70. Crukshank SH, Stoelk EM. Surgical control of pelvic hemorrhage: bilateral hypogastric artery ligation and method of ovarian artery ligation. Southampt Med J 1985;78:539–43.
71. Nizard J, Barrinque L, Frydman R, et al. Fertility and pregnancy outcomes following hypogastric artery ligation for severe post-partum haemorrhage. Humanit Rep 2003;18:844–8.
72. Heaston DK, Mineau DE, Brown BJ, et al. Transcatheter arterial embolization for control of persistent massive puerperal hemorrhage after bilateral surgical hypogastric artery ligation. AJR Am J Roentgenol 1979;133:152–4.
73. Kunstlinger F, Brunelle F, Chaumont P, et al. Vascular occlusive agents. AJR 1981; 136:151–6.
74. Chou MM, Hwang JI, Tseng JJ, et al. Internal iliac artery embolization before hysterectomy for placenta accreta. J Vasc Interv Radiol 2003;14:1195–9.
75. Vedantham S, Goodwin SC, McLucas B, et al. Uterine artery embolization: an underused method of controlling pelvic hemorrhage. Am J Obstet Gynecol 1997; 176:938–48.
76. Doumouchtsis SK, Papageorghiou AT, Arulkumaran S. Systematic review of conservative management of postpartum hemorrhage: what to do when medical treatment fails. Obstet Gynecol Surv 2007;62:540–7.
77. Vegas G, Illescas T, Munoz M, et al. Selective pelvic arterial embolization in the management of obstetric hemorrhage. Eur J Obstet Gynecol Reprod Biol 2006; 127:68–72.
78. Cordonnier C, Ha-Vien DE, Depret S, et al. Foetal growth restriction in the next pregnancy after uterine artery embolisation for post-partum haemorrhage. Eur J Obstet Gynecol Reprod Biol 2002;103:183–4.
79. Salomon LJ, deTayrac R, Castaigne-Meary V, et al. Fertility and pregnancy outcome following pelvic arterial embolization for severe post-partum haemorrhage: a cohort study. Hum Reprod 2003;18:849–52.
80. Levine AB, Kuhlman K, Bonn J. Placenta accreta: comparison of cases managed with and without pelvic artery balloon catheters. J Matern Fetal Med 1999;8: 173–6.
81. Dubois J, Garel L, Grignon A, et al. Placenta percreta: balloon occlusion and embolization of the internal iliac arteries to reduce intraoperative blood losses. Am J Obstet Gynecol 1997;176:723–6.
82. Shrivastava V, Nageotte M, Major C, et al. Case-control comparison of cesarean hysterectomy with and without prophylactic placement of intravascular balloon catheters for placenta accreta. Am J Obstet Gynecol 2007;197:402e1–5.
83. Miura F, Takada T, Ochiai T, et al. Aortic occlusion balloon catheter technique is useful for uncontrollable massive intraabdominal bleeding after hepato-pancreato-biliary surgery. J Gastrointest Surg 2006;10:519–22.

Minimizing Perinatal Neurologic Injury at Term: Is Cesarean Section the Answer?

Russell Miller, MD[a],*, Richard Depp, MD[b]

KEYWORDS

• Cesarean section • Emergency cesarean section
• Neonatal encephalopathy • Cerebral palsy • 30-minute rule

The last half-century has witnessed a dramatic increase in cesarean section use and an accompanying exaggeration of its benefits. In 2005, a record 30.2% of births in the United States were by cesarean delivery, representing a 46% rise since 1006.[1] Among these births, a trend appears to exist toward an increasing proportion of cesarean deliveries because of nonreassuring fetal heart status (NRFHS).[2-4] This national prevalence of cesarean delivery for NRFHS is substantial: pooled data from 19 observational studies published between 1992 and 2000 with more than 1000 patients each indicate that it may represent 2.6% of all deliveries.[2,3] However, these relative and absolute increases in cesarean section for presumed fetal neuroprotective benefit havo not been accompanied by a concomitant improvement in perinatal neurologic outcomes, as exhibited by the incidence of cerebral palsy (CP).[5-8] Over the last tew decades, the prevalence of CP among term deliveries has remained constant, if not slightly increased, at 2.0 per 1000 live births.[6]

Although no compelling proof exists of a neuroprotective benefit from an expedited cesarean delivery for NRFHS, by applying arbitrary standards for timely intervention to cases involving potentially significant fetal hypoxia, obstetricians may be placing multiple parties at considerable risk without comparable chance for reward. Fetuses are placed at increased risk for iatrogenic trauma as a result of emergent cesarean delivery.[9-11] Mothers undergoing emergency cesarean delivery face an increased risk for intraoperative complications, including hemorrhage, blood transfusion, and genitourinary injury,[9,12-14] and for delayed complications, such as posttraumatic stress disorder.[15] Lastly, although not manifest in the same direct physical or psychologic sense, the risk to the obstetric community in this setting may be just as real.

a Division of Maternal Fetal Medicine, Department of Obstetrics and Gynecology, Columbia University Medical Center, 622 West 168th Street, PH 16-66, New York, NY 10032, USA
b Drexel University College of Medicine, Philadelphia, PA, USA
* Corresponding author.
E-mail address: rsm20@columbia.edu (R. Miller)

Clin Perinatol 35 (2008) 549–559
doi:10.1016/j.clp.2008.07.005
0095-5108/08/$ – see front matter © 2008 Elsevier Inc. All rights reserved.
perinatology.theclinics.com

Through its application of delivery practices that are not substantiated by available evidence,[16] the obstetric community may be placing its patients at unnecessary risk by propagating clinical practices that are inherently unreasonable.

This article evaluates the role of cesarean delivery at term as a strategy for minimizing perinatal neurologic injury in the form of neonatal encephalopathy (NNE) or subsequent CP. The issue will be framed within the current medicolegal and public climate before it is explored on a pathophysiologic and clinical level. The history and evidence supporting contemporary guidelines of obstetric care for fetal neuroprotective benefit are analyzed, and alterative care strategies are proposed.

MEDICOLEGAL CONTEXT

Failure to extricate a fetus expeditiously from an inhospitable intrauterine environment is a common allegation in medical negligence claims involving neurologically impaired neonates. Concerns regarding fetal monitoring interpretation, the appropriateness of timing, and the route of delivery are usually at the heart of allegations of substandard intrapartum care.[17] When negligence and causation are established, they can be associated with a staggering cost: in 2005, the median award in the United States for "medical negligence in child birth cases" was $2.5 million.[18]

Although obstetric care is seldom the cause of profound neonatal injury, the cumulative risk for medical malpractice litigation to practicing obstetricians is great. In its most recent 2006 Survey on Professional Liability, the American College of Obstetricians and Gynecologists (ACOG) reported that 89.2% of 10,659 respondents indicated they had experienced at least one professional liability claim filed against them during their professional careers, with an average of 2.62 claims per obstetrician-gynecologist.[19] Among obstetric claims, the most common primary claim involved allegations of a neurologically impaired infant, in 30.8% of cases.[19]

Given this risk for professional liability claims, practicing obstetricians may be influenced to practice defensive medicine, defined as an alteration of previously standard practice patterns to avoid potential litigation. In the aforementioned survey, 64.6% of respondents reported having made one or more changes to their practice because of fear of litigation, with 37.1% of respondents reporting that they altered obstetric practices, increasing the number of cesarean sections performed.[19] In a 1997 analytic investigation into the existence of defensive medicine in New York State, 58,441 obstetric deliveries were reviewed and compared with cumulative obstetric malpractice suits, which were considered a proxy for physician fear of malpractice.[20] Of an overall cesarean section rate of 27.6%, "fear of malpractice" was estimated to account for 6.6 percentage points, further suggesting an influence of defensive medicine on obstetric practices.

With a perceived societal "zero tolerance" for imperfect outcomes in a field where outcomes cannot be guaranteed (yet the CP rate predictable at approximately 2 per 1000 live deliveries), it is understandable that some obstetricians have resorted to defensive practice strategies. However, no evidence exists that altering practice to increase cesarean delivery rates will successfully prevent cases of intrapartum neurologic injury. A 2002 analysis by Bailit and colleagues[21] compared predicted risk-adjusted hospital primary cesarean delivery rates and rates of neonatal asphyxia with actual cesarean delivery rates between 1995 and 1996 across Washington state hospitals. The investigators found that the highest risk for asphyxia was experienced at institutions where cesarean deliveries performed exceeded predicted cesarean deliveries, suggesting that overall cesarean delivery rate is not a satisfactory marker for quality of obstetric care or necessarily protective against adverse neonatal outcomes.

PUBLIC AWARENESS

Although multimillion dollar jury findings may suggest otherwise, limited data indicate mixed public awareness regarding the pathogenesis of CP and its preventability by cesarean delivery. In 2002, Feldman-Winter and colleagues[22] published the results of a survey of 100 randomly sampled adults selected from the waiting room of a suburban ambulatory pediatrics office in New Jersey. Participants were asked questions regarding their general perceptions of CP. Most study participants were educated, middle to upper-middle class, and married. Although 35.6% of respondents agreed with the statement that CP is "usually due to a birth injury associated with problems during labor and delivery," only 8.9% agreed that CP "can be prevented by cesarean section." These beliefs may not accurately represent those held by other less socio-economically advantaged groups; however, the results demonstrated that most survey respondents were aware of a lack of neuroprotective benefit to cesarean delivery. The role of educational outreach efforts and media publicity in highlighting this particular issue remains unexplored to date.

THE CAUSE AND TIMING OF NEONATAL ENCEPHALOPATHY AND CEREBRAL PALSY

To best understand the minimal impact that cesarean delivery may have on perinatal neurologic outcomes requires an appreciation of the relationship, cause, and timing between intrapartum hypoxic-ischemic injury, NNE, and resultant CP. According to the ACOG Task Force[23] on NNE and CP, NNE is defined in term and near-term infants as "a constellation of findings to include a combination of abnormal consciousness, tone and reflexes, feeding, respiration, or seizures and can result from myriad conditions." A few, perhaps as few as 4%, of cases of moderate and severe NNE are believed to be attributable to hypoxia incurred solely during the intrapartum period, explaining the estimated low overall prevalence of NNE due to intrapartum hypoxia (1.6 per 10,000 live births).[23-25] NNE does not always progress to permanent neurologic impairment. However, when permanent disability develops, it is manifest as CP, a nonprogressive deficiency of central neuromotor function usually characterized by abnormal movement and posture. For a case of CP to be attributed accurately to an antecedent intrapartum hypoxic-ischemic injury, it first must necessarily progress through NNE of hypoxic-ischemic origin.[23] This sequence of causal events linking hypoxic-ischemic insult to NNE and subsequent CP is important to consider when evaluating possible perinatal neuroprotective strategies.

In the 1998 West Australian case-control study, Badawi and colleagues[24,25] evaluated antenatal and intrapartum risk factors for NNE in 164 term infants who had moderate or severe NNE compared with 400 randomly selected controls. The investigators determined a birth prevalence for moderate or severe NNE of 3.8 per 1000 term live births. Sixty-nine percent of cases possessed no evidence of adverse intrapartum events, 24% of cases had antepartum and intrapartum risk factors, and 5% of cases had only intrapartum risk factors identified. A follow-up study of outcomes at 5 years in an expanded cohort of cases demonstrated a 13% rate of CP among survivors of moderate or severe NNE.[26] When compared with total cases of CP in Western Australia over the same study period, CP following NNE comprised only 24% of total cases of term CP.

Other literature supports only a limited contribution of intrapartum hypoxic-ischemic injury to the rare outcome of term CP. In 2006, Stribjis and colleagues[27] reviewed 213 cases of CP from a single Australian tertiary care center over an 18-year period. Major antenatal or postnatal CP-related pathologies were identified in 98.1% of cases. Among 46 term deliveries, an isolated acute intrapartum hypoxic-ischemic event was deemed likely in only 2 instances (4.3%). None of the term cases met all four of the ACOG/American Academy of Pediatrics (AAP) essential criteria for a hypoxic-ischemic event to be a possible cause of CP. In fact, the 2 cases suspected to be due to an intrapartum insult had blood gas results that were inconsistent with a severe metabolic academia. Therefore, based on these data, cesarean section, emergent or otherwise, should not be expected to prevent most cases of term CP, because most cases lack an intrapartum basis.

In the uncommon instance when intrapartum hypoxic-ischemic injury does contribute to neurologic injury, the pathway begins with impaired fetal cerebral blood flow following interrupted placental circulatory or gas exchange.[28,29] The resulting hypoxemia initiates a state of anaerobic metabolism, which eventually causes a severe metabolic academia that triggers a series of disruptive events at the cellular level. It is unclear how underlying fetal susceptibility interacts with duration or severity of hypoxia to determine whether an in utero insult will progress to permanent neurologic injury. Furthermore, the precise timing of this injury can be difficult to pinpoint on a case-by-case basis. Retrospective use of blood markers and algorithms for timing hypoxic injury are often inaccurate and dependent on potentially inappropriate assumptions.[30,31] And, as the following section discusses, electronic fetal heart rate monitoring (EFM) interpretation, the current standard for intrapartum fetal assessment, is not prospectively reliable at predicting the timing of hypoxic-ischemic insults for the accurate identification of which deliveries, if any, might benefit from immediate pregnancy interruption by emergent cesarean section.

Further detracting from claims that properly timed cesarean deliveries might decrease the incidence of term CP, data indicate that intrauterine infection is a significant risk factor for CP, and a more common cause for CP than hypoxic-ischemic injury. In 1997, Grether and Nelson[32] demonstrated a strong association between spastic CP and maternal temperature, chorioamnionitis, and histologic evidence of infection among infants of normal birth weight. They concluded that maternal infection poses significant risk to the developing fetus, potentially accounting for 12% of total cases of spastic CP, including 19% of unexplained cases. In a subsequent 2003 case-control investigation involving term and near-term infants, Wu and colleagues[33] demonstrated that chorioamnionitis was an independent risk factor for neurologic injury present in 14% of CP cases. In this study, a significant association between intrauterine infection and CP persisted in 6% of cases that were attributed to hypoxic-ischemic injury.

The pathophysiologic cascade linking chorioamnionitis to neurologic injury is currently a topic of investigation but it involves some combination of elevated levels of circulating proinflammatory fetal cytokines, inflammatory changes in placental membranes leading to placental hypoperfusion, pyrexia-induced neurologic injury, and direct infection of the fetal brain.[33–36] Given that these represent different mechanisms for fetal tissue injury than hypoxia-ischemia, it is unreasonable to expect intrapartum fetal monitoring technologies intended to identify hypoxic-ischemia (such as electronic fetal monitoring) to also identify cases of infection-induced fetal injury. Furthermore, it is unclear what benefit, if any, urgent cesarean delivery has in diminishing the risk for CP once clinical or subclinical intrauterine infection has occurred.

NONREASSURING FETAL HEART STATUS

Complementing a skyrocketing cesarean delivery rate, EFM is another intervention intended to improve pregnancy outcomes that has been widely integrated into standard obstetric practice without yielding any evidence to support a reduction in CP following term deliveries or otherwise.[37–40] Despite lackluster efficacy in the prediction of outcomes other than in utero demise, EFM is the predominant form of intrapartum fetal surveillance in the United States.

As noted in the 2005 ACOG Practice Bulletin[40] on FHR monitoring, obstetricians exhibit considerable intra- and interobserver variability when interpreting FHR patterns. In addition to inconsistent and subjective assessments, the significance of physician-established FHR patterns remains incompletely understood. In the 1997 National Institute of Child Health and Human Development Research Planning Workshop[41] publication on research guidelines for fetal heart rate (FHR) pattern interpretation, workshop participants cited an inability to reach consensus regarding precise guidelines for clinical management using FHR patterns. Participants agreed on patterns characteristic of "normal" FHR tracings, and patterns predictive of "current or impending fetal asphyxia so severe that the fetus is at risk for neurologic and other fetal damage, or death." Inclusion in this latter group of grossly abnormal patterns required the presence of recurrent late or variable decelerations or substantial bradycardia, and absent variability. However, workshop contributors acknowledged the presence of a third large group of intermediate FHR patterns that did not clearly fall into the absolutely normal or abnormal groups, and for which no consensus for management could be reached.

Partly owing to the above limitations, although biologically an attractive theory, the correlation between ominous FHR patterns and evolving fetal hypoxic-ischemic injury is tenuous. In 1996, Nelson and colleagues[42] demonstrated that although specific EFM patterns were associated with an increased risk for CP, use of these abnormal patterns to predict cases of CP was associated with an "extremely high" false-positive rate, estimated at 99.8%. Clark and Hankins[38] further critiqued the value of FHR monitoring in 2003, stating that, "A test leading to an unnecessary major abdominal operation in more than 99.5% of cases should be regarded by the medical community as absurd at best." Despite the reported flaws of EFM, the relative and absolute numbers of cesarean deliveries performed for NRFHS continue to rise.

THE "30-MINUTE RULE"

Although It is evident that EFM lacks predictive value as a clinical tool, in some instances, an FHR pattern or obstetric emergency (ie, a cord prolapse) warrant expeditious delivery. Under most circumstances, emergency cesarean delivery in such scenarios is considered to fall under the "30-minute rule." As defined in guidelines published by ACOG and the AAP,[16] "hospitals should have the capability of performing a cesarean delivery within 30 minutes of the decision to operate." However, this delivery guideline can be challenging to meet in everyday practice on the average labor unit. Many, if not all, institutions are likely to experience difficulty in consistently adhering to a policy of a 30-minute decision-to-delivery interval (DDI).

The controversial value of the "30-minute rule" is poorly founded and the rule is of uncertain benefit. The "30-minute rule" is based on little more than a few primate studies correlating length of asphyxia with brain injury, and consensus opinion.[16,29,43–45] As this section details, human data fail to support the "30-minute rule."[45–52] The "30-minute rule" therefore may not represent a true cutoff for achieving improved perinatal outcomes, and its continued support may not be justified.

Schauberger and colleagues[45] published the first modern investigation of DDI as it relates to the "30-minute rule." Between 1985 and 1991, the investigators retrospectively identified 75 emergency cesarean sections occurring at a single tertiary-care hospital. Indications for deliveries included "fetal distress," cord prolapse, and maternal hemorrhage. Two control groups matched for gestational age and parity were created; the first control group consisted of subjects undergoing nonemergent intrapartum cesarean deliveries, and the second group consisted of subjects undergoing cesarean delivery in the absence of labor.

Overall, 63% of deliveries in the emergency cesarean group were started within 30 minutes of decision time. Within this group, a significantly greater number of neonates with DDI less than 30 minutes had 5-minute Apgar scores under six when compared with those with DDI greater than 30 minutes (23% versus 3.6%, P = .02). However, significant differences were also not observed in neonatal ICU (NICU) admission rates, durations of NICU stay, rates of "acidotic" arterial cord pH (defined as pH<7.1), and mean cord pH. Clinical end points such as NNE and CP were not commented on in this study.

When emergent and nonemergent deliveries were compared, decreased Apgar scores at 1 and 5 minutes were observed following emergency deliveries. Otherwise, "acidotic" arterial cord pH rates, NICU admission rates, durations of NICU stays, and neonatal mortality were not different between the groups. Two neonatal lacerations occurred following emergency cesarean deliveries; each had a DDI less than 30 minutes. Maternal morbidities were not different between the groups. Based on these data, the investigators questioned whether the "30-minute rule" has a beneficial effect on neonatal outcomes.

Tuffnell and colleagues[46] evaluated DDI in the setting of urgent cesarean sections performed at a single institution in the United Kingdom. Over a 4-year period beginning in 1993, three 3-month audits were conducted, followed by a 32-month continuous audit. The institutional rate of emergency cesarean delivery over the audit period ranged from 9% to 12%. The investigators identified 721 emergency cesarean deliveries over the continuous audit period, 478 (66.3%) of which had a DDI less than 30 minutes. Among the subset of deliveries at 36 weeks or greater gestational age, no differences existed in special care admissions when deliveries were stratified by 30-minute DDI cutoff. A single case of hypoxic-ischemic NNE was observed in the setting of a placental abruption at an unreported gestational age; in this case, the DDI was 20 minutes. The investigators concluded that a 30-minute standard was not being consistently achieved in their audits, but that these failures were not associated with increased neonatal morbidities.

MacKenzie and Cooke[47,51] prospectively evaluated DDI as it related to nonelective cesarean deliveries occurring during calendar year 1996 at a single institution in the United Kingdom. In this study, "emergency" cesarean sections were defined as decisions to proceed with cesarean delivery based on intrapartum clinical diagnoses including fetal distress, labor dystocia, and maternal indications. "Emergency" deliveries were distinguished from "crash" deliveries (impending fetal death, such as a cord prolapse or uterine rupture, or serious maternal compromise anticipated); "urgent" deliveries (decision made during the 24 hours before delivery because of deteriorating fetal or maternal status before labor onset); and "pre-empted" deliveries (decision made more than 24 hours before the onset of spontaneous labor or membrane rupture).

Three hundred eighty-five "emergency" deliveries with accompanying cord arterial pH results were identified, of which "fetal distress" was the primary documented clinical indication in 126 cases (32.7%). Three hundred thirty (86%) of this group had a documented DDI. Overall, fewer than 40% of "emergency" deliveries due to "fetal distress" with known DDI were performed within 30 minutes of the decision to operate. "Emergency" deliveries due to "fetal distress" had a significantly shorter DDI (mean 42.9 minutes) than those without "distress" (mean 71.1 minutes). DDI for "emergency" deliveries fell between a mean DDI of 27.4 minutes for "crash" deliveries and 124.7 minutes for "urgent" deliveries.

As DDI lengthened within the "emergency" cesarean section group, a surprising "trend of improved cord arterial pH values with more prolonged delivery times with and without fetal distress" occurred.[47] Although a trend toward greater academia with shorter DDI may suggest physicians' abilities to select those cases requiring more expeditious delivery, this study was not designed to address this hypothesis directly. Regardless of the cause, MacKenzie and Cooke demonstrated that although a DDI less than 30 minutes was not achieved in most of the "emergency" deliveries observed in their cohort, delays were not associated with an adverse influence on cord gas results.

Holcroft and colleagues[48] evaluated the relationship between umbilical artery pH and DDI in the setting of "emergent" and "urgent" cesarean sections due to NRFHS at a single institution. On retrospective chart summary and EFM review, three maternal-fetal medicine specialists blinded to neonatal outcomes classified cesarean deliveries as either "emergent" (requiring delivery as soon as possible) or "urgent" (delivery could wait up to 30 minutes). When a unanimous opinion could not be reached, a majority decision was used to classify cases. Of 117 subjects included, 34 cases were determined to be emergent and 83 urgent. A kappa of 0.35 suggested fair-to-moderate agreement between chart reviewers.

In the emergent group, the DDI was 14 minutes shorter in the emergency group (mean 23 ± 15.3 minutes) when compared with the "urgent" group (mean 36.7 ± 14.9 minutes, $P < .001$). A significant relationship existed between shorter DDI and cases with worse cord umbilical artery pH and base excess results. Overall, no abrupt deterioration in cord gas results occurred after 30 minutes, and most neonates delivered after this cutoff had normal cord gas results. Of 13 cases with either an umbilical artery pH less than 7.0 or base excess less than 12 mmol/L, the DDI was 24.7 ± 14.6 minutes (with a range of 6 to 50 minutes). Three (23%) of these cases were classified as urgent deliveries. No cases of neonatal seizures or periventricular leukoencephalomalacia occurred. The delivery groups showed no difference in the rate of intraventricular hemorrhage, and this complication was likely related to preterm deliveries within each group. NNE and CP were not specifically noted as outcomes in this study.

The case review system used in this study had sensitivity and specificity of 77%, positive predictive value of 29%, and negative predictive value of 96% for the prediction of an umbilical artery pH less than 7.0 or base excess less than 12 mmol/L. The investigators concluded that their findings reflected a professional imprecision in the diagnosis of NRFHS, as previously highlighted by the 1997 NICHD consensus statement, and stated that normal outcomes should therefore be expected even when the DDI exceeds 30 minutes.

Thomas and colleagues[52] published the results of a national cross-sectional survey investigating the value of DDI in emergency cesarean sections. Over a 3-month period in the year 2000, deliveries were audited across maternity units in England and Wales. DDI, neonatal outcomes (Apgar scores and stillbirth diagnoses), and maternal outcomes were collected.

Overall, 17,780 singleton births emergency cesarean deliveries were identified. The investigators found no difference in neonatal or maternal outcomes when deliveries with DDI less than 30 minutes were compared with those with DDI between 31 and 75 minutes. However, after 75 minutes, 5-minute Apgar scores under seven increased by 80%, and maternal care requirements increased by 60%. The investigators concluded that, although their data could not substantiate benefit to a 30-minute delivery requirement, a DDI greater than 75 minutes may be associated with poorer neonatal and maternal outcomes and should be avoided.

Lastly, Bloom and colleagues[50] conducted a secondary analysis of the Maternal-Fetal Medicine Network's cesarean delivery registry investigating relationships between decision-to-incision interval (DII) and maternal and neonatal outcomes following emergency deliveries. Emergency deliveries involved diagnoses of cord prolapse, placental abruption, placenta previa with hemorrhage, NRFHS, and uterine rupture.

From this prospective cohort, 2808 emergency deliveries were identified. Of these, 65% of emergency deliveries had a DII of 30 minutes or less. Maternal complications were not different based on a 30-minute cutoff. Umbilical artery pH less than 7.0 and neonatal intubation requirements were both higher in the subset of deliveries occurring within 30 minutes of the decision to operate. In those deliveries with a DII greater than 30 minutes, 95% of neonates did not experience evidence of newborn compromise. Rates of hypoxic-ischemic encephalopathy were similar between groups stratified by 30-minute DII, with 12/1814 (0.7%) in the under group and 5/994 (0.5%) in the over group ($P = .61$).

Although methodologic differences limit formal comparisons among the studies summarized above, a review of this collected literature reveals two consistent findings. The first is that medical centers in the United States and United Kingdom have difficulty applying a "30-minute rule" to a substantial proportion of emergency cesarean deliveries. The second is that a DDI greater than 30 minutes is not associated with an increased rate of adverse neonatal outcomes. On the contrary, the trend noted in several investigations is that markers for adverse neonatal outcomes (cord gas results, Apgar scores) appear to worsen as DDI shortens. This finding may be explained by physicians' abilities to select and promptly deliver those cases at highest risk for compromise from cases requiring less rapid intervention. In support of this theory, Kolas and colleagues[49] identified 1511 emergency cesarean deliveries from a Norwegian birth registry to determine factors that influence DDI. Variance in DDI was mainly explained by selected indications for emergency cesarean section, including placental abruption, cord prolapse, and NRFHS.

"Emergency" cesarean section is a nonspecific term with a sole requirement of a perceived immediate need for an operative pregnancy interruption. This term does not describe the underlying indication for delivery. Because considerable heterogeneity exists with respect to indications for "emergency" cesarean delivery, standards for timely intervention should be tailored according to the underlying cause of the pregnancy disturbance and the associated likelihood that a given delay to delivery will lead to neonatal compromise. Until indication-specific data are available, decisions regarding delivery timing may be best left to the discretion of the delivering obstetrician, and not covered under a blanket 30-minute delivery policy.

SUMMARY

Despite advances in obstetric and neonatal care, the last several decades have not witnessed an improvement in the prediction or prevention of term CP. Obstetric interventions such as EFM and cesarean delivery, although biologically plausible as intervention strategies, do not improve perinatal outcomes in clinical practice. In reaction to mounting medicolegal pressure, obstetricians continue to increase the number of cesarean deliveries they perform as a form of defensive medicine, despite evidence that this practice is not associated with improved perinatal outcomes.

The current standard for expeditious delivery in a case of potential fetal compromise is described by the "30-minute rule." Initially derived from limited data, the "30-minute" rule appears to represent an invalid absolute threshold for obstetric intervention. This standard is difficult to meet regularly in clinical practice, yet failure to achieve it is not associated with an increase in adverse neonatal outcomes unless it is greatly exceeded in time. Obstetricians' determinations of the need for expedited delivery may be a preferable guide for appropriate delivery timing.

REFERENCES

1. Hamilton BE, Minino AM, Martin JA, et al. Annual summary of vital statistics: 2005. Pediatrics 2007;119(2):345–60.
2. Chauhan SP, Magann EF, Scott JR, et al. Cesarean delivery for fetal distress: rate and risk factors. Obstet Gynecol Surv 2003;58(5):337–50.
3. Gregory KD, Curtin SC, Taffel SM, et al. Changes in indications for cesarean delivery: United States, 1985 and 1994. Am J Public Health 1998;88(9):1384–7.
4. Joseph KS, Young DC, Dodds L, et al. Changes in maternal characteristics and obstetric practice and recent increases in primary cesarean delivery. Obstet Gynecol 2003;102(4):791–800.
5. Nelson KB. The epidemiology of cerebral palsy in term infants. Ment Retard Dev Disabil Res Rev 2002;8(3):146–50.
6. Winter S, Autry A, Boyle C, et al. Trends in the prevalence of cerebral palsy in a population-based study. Pediatrics 2002;110(6):1220–5.
7. Colver AF, Gibson M, Hey EN, et al. Increasing rates of cerebral palsy across the severity spectrum in north-east England 1964–1993. The North of England Collaborative Cerebral Palsy Survey. Arch Dis Child Fetal Neonatal Ed 2000;83(1): F7–12.
8. Wu YW, Croon LA, Shah SJ, et al. Cerebral palsy in a term population: risk factors and neuroimaging findings. Pediatrics 2006;118(2):690–7.
9. Hager RM, Daltveit AK, Hofoss D, et al. Complications of cesarean deliveries: rates and risk factors. Am J Obstet Gynecol 2004;190(2):428–34.
10. Dessole S, Cosmi E, Balata A, et al. Accidental fetal lacerations during cesarean delivery: experience in an Italian level III university hospital. Am J Obstet Gynecol 2004;191(5):1673–7.
11. Alexander JM, Leveno KJ, Hauth J, et al. Fetal injury associated with cesarean delivery. Obstet Gynecol 2006;108(4):885–90.
12. van Ham MA, van Dongen PW, Mulder J. Maternal consequences of caesarean section. A retrospective study of intra-operative and postoperative maternal complications of caesarean section during a 10-year period. Eur J Obstet Gynecol Reprod Biol 1997;74(1):1–6.
13. Rajasekar D, Hall M. Urinary tract injuries during obstetric intervention. Br J Obstet Gynaecol 1997;104(6):731–4.
14. Phipps MG, Watabe B, Clemons JL, et al. Risk factors for bladder injury during cesarean delivery. Obstet Gynecol 2005;105(1):156–60.
15. Olde E, van der Hart O, Kleber R, et al. Posttraumatic stress following childbirth: a review. Clin Psychol Rev 2006;26(1):1–16.
16. American Academy of Pediatrics, American College of Obstetricians and Gynecologists. Intrapartum and postpartum care of women. Guidelines for perinatal care. 5th edition. Elk Grove Village (IL): AAP; 2002. Washington, DC: ACOG: AAP/ACOG.
17. Cohen WR, Schifrin BS. Medical negligence lawsuits relating to labor and delivery. Clin Perinatol 2007;34(2):345–60, vii–viii.
18. Thomas C, editor. Jury verdict research: current award trends in personal injury. 46th edition. Horsham (PA): LRP Publications; 2007.

19. Wilson N, Strunk AL. Overview of the 2006 ACOG survey on professional liability. ACOG Clinical Review 2007;12(2):1, 13–6.
20. Tussing AD, Wojtowycz MA. Malpractice, defensive medicine, and obstetric behavior. Med Care 1997;35(2):172–91.
21. Bailit JL, Garrett JM, Miller WC, et al. Hospital primary cesarean delivery rates and the risk of poor neonatal outcomes. Am J Obstet Gynecol 2002;187(3): 721–7.
22. Feldman-Winter LB, Krueger CJ, Neyhart JM, et al. Public perceptions of cerebral palsy. J Am Osteopath Assoc 2002;102(9):471–5.
23. American College of Obstetricians and Gynecologists' Task Force on Neonatal Encephalopathy and Cerebral Palsy, American College of Obstetricians and Gynecologists, American Academy of Pediatrics. Neonatal encephalopathy and cerebral palsy: defining the pathogenesis and pathophysiology. 94th edition. Washington, DC: ACOG; 2003.
24. Badawi N, Kurinczuk JJ, Keogh JM, et al. Antepartum risk factors for newborn encephalopathy: the Western Australian case-control study. BMJ 1998; 317(7172):1549–53.
25. Badawi N, Kurinczuk JJ, Keogh JM, et al. Intrapartum risk factors for newborn encephalopathy: the Western Australian case-control study. BMJ 1998;317(7172): 1554–8.
26. Badawi N, Felix JF, Kurinczuk JJ, et al. Cerebral palsy following term newborn encephalopathy: a population-based study. Dev Med Child Neurol 2005;47(5): 293–8.
27. Strijbis EM, Oudman I, van Essen P, et al. Cerebral palsy and the application of the international criteria for acute intrapartum hypoxia. Obstet Gynecol 2006; 107(6):1357–65.
28. Shalak L, Perlman JM. Hypoxic-ischemic brain injury in the term infant-current concepts. Early Hum Dev 2004;80(2):125–41.
29. Myers RE. Two patterns of perinatal brain damage and their conditions of occurrence. Am J Obstet Gynecol 1972;112(2):246–76.
30. Naeye RL, Lin HM. Determination of the timing of fetal brain damage from hypoxemia-ischemia. Am J Obstet Gynecol 2001;184(2):217–24.
31. Ross MG, Gala R. Use of umbilical artery base excess: algorithm for the timing of hypoxic injury. Am J Obstet Gynecol 2002;187(1):1–9.
32. Grether JK, Nelson KB. Maternal infection and cerebral palsy in infants of normal birth weight. JAMA 1997;278(3):207–11.
33. Wu YW, Escobar GJ, Grether JK, et al. Chorioamnionitis and cerebral palsy in term and near-term infants. JAMA 2003;290(20):2677–84.
34. Romero R, Espinoza J, Goncalves LF, et al. The role of inflammation and infection in preterm birth. Semin Reprod Med 2007;25(1):21–39.
35. Pacora P, Chaiworapongsa T, Maymon E, et al. Funisitis and chorionic vasculitis: the histological counterpart of the fetal inflammatory response syndrome. J Matern Fetal Neonatal Med 2002;11(1):18–25.
36. Yoon BH, Romero R, Park JS, et al. Fetal exposure to an intra-amniotic inflammation and the development of cerebral palsy at the age of three years. Am J Obstet Gynecol 2000;182(3):675–81.
37. Parer JT, King T. Fetal heart rate monitoring: is it salvageable? Am J Obstet Gynecol 2000;182(4):982–7.
38. Clark SL, Hankins GD. Temporal and demographic trends in cerebral palsy–fact and fiction. Am J Obstet Gynecol 2003;188(3):628–33.

39. Freeman RK. Problems with intrapartum fetal heart rate monitoring interpretation and patient management. Obstet Gynecol 2002;100(4):813–26.

40. ACOG practice bulletin. Clinical management guidelines for obstetrician-gynecologists, number 70, December 2005 (replaces practice bulletin number 62, May 2005). Intrapartum fetal heart rate monitoring. Obstet Gynecol 2005; 106(6):1453–60.

41. National Institute of Child Health and Human Development Research Planning Workshop. Electronic fetal heart rate monitoring: research guidelines for interpretation. Am J Obstet Gynecol 1997;177(6):1385–90.

42. Nelson KB, Dambrosia JM, Ting TY, et al. Uncertain value of electronic fetal monitoring in predicting cerebral palsy. N Engl J Med 1996;334(10):613–8.

43. Myers RE, Beard R, Adamsons K. Brain swelling in the newborn rhesus monkey following prolonged partial asphyxia. Neurology 1969;19(10):1012–8.

44. Adamsons K, Myers RE. Late decelerations and brain tolerance of the fetal monkey to intrapartum asphyxia. Am J Obstet Gynecol 1977;128(8):893–900.

45. Schauberger CW, Rooney BL, Beguin EA, et al. Evaluating the thirty minute interval in emergency cesarean sections. J Am Coll Surg 1994;179(2):151–5.

46. Tuffnell DJ, Wilkinson K, Beresford N. Interval between decision and delivery by caesarean section-are current standards achievable? Observational case series. BMJ 2001;322(7298):1330–3.

47. MacKenzie IZ, Cooke I. Prospective 12 month study of 30 minute decision to delivery intervals for "emergency" caesarean section. BMJ 2001;322(7298):1334–5.

48. Holcroft CJ, Graham EM, Aina-Mumuney A, et al. Cord gas analysis, decision-to-delivery interval, and the 30-minute rule for emergency cesareans. J Perinatol 2005;25(4):229–35.

49. Kolas T, Hofoss D, Oian P. Predictions for the decision-to-delivery interval for emergency cesarean sections in Norway. Acta Obstet Gynecol Scand 2006; 85(5):561–6.

50. Bloom SL, Leveno KJ, Spong CY, et al. Decision-to-incision times and maternal and infant outcomes. Obstet Gynecol 2006;108(1):6–11.

51. MacKenzie IZ, Cooke I. What is a reasonable time from decision-to-delivery by caesarean section? Evidence from 415 deliveries. BJOG 2002;109(5):498–504.

52. Thomas J, Paranjothy S, James D. National cross sectional survey to determine whether the decision to delivery interval is critical in emergency caesarean section. BMJ 2004;328(7441):665–9.

Effect of Placental Transfusion on the Blood Volume and Clinical Outcome of Infants Born by Cesarean Section

Venkatakrishna Kakkilaya, MD, MBBS, Arun K. Pramanik, MD, MBBS*,
Hassan Ibrahim, MD, MBBCH, Sameh Hussein, MD, MBBCH

KEYWORDS

- Placental transfusion • Blood volume
- Newborn infants • Cesarean section
- Umbilical cord clamping • Blood transfusion

The blood volume of a term fetus is approximately 70 mL/kg. The placenta contains 45 mL/kg of blood, making the total fetoplacental volume 115 mL/kg. Premature infants have larger placenta when compared with term neonates; therefore, the fetoplacental volume is 150 mL at 26 weeks' gestation. The fetoplacental blood volume decreases with increasing gestation. The newborn infant's blood volume at birth is dependent on the transfer of blood between the placenta and fetus.[1] A redistribution of blood between the fetus and placenta results from an imbalance of umbilical arterial and venous blood flow. A relative increase in umbilical arterial blood flow causes loss to fetal blood into the placenta, whereas a relative increase in umbilical venous blood flow results in the fetus gaining blood from the placenta. According to Poiseuille's law, blood flow through a vessel increases directly with the pressure gradient and the fourth power of the vessel diameter. Transfusion of blood from the placenta to the fetus occurs as a result of umbilical arterial vasodilatation or an increase in the pressure gradient between the arteries and the umbilical vein. Transfusion of blood from the placenta to the fetus is to be expected when the diameter of the umbilical vein increases or the pressure gradient between the umbilical vein and central veins in the fetus increases.[1]

When the umbilical cord is clamped soon after birth, the infant's blood volume is similar to its in utero volume. In contrast, a delay in clamping the umbilical cord may

Louisiana State University Health Sciences Center, 1501 Kings Highway, P.O. Box 33932, Shreveport, LA 71130, USA
* Corresponding author.
E-mail address: aprama@lsuhsc.edu (A.K. Pramanik).

Clin Perinatol 35 (2008) 561–570
doi:10.1016/j.clp.2008.07.002
0095-5108/08/$ – see front matter © 2008 Elsevier Inc. All rights reserved.

perinatology.theclinics.com

result in transfer of additional blood to the newborn infant during cesarean section and vaginal deliveries.[2–11] Several factors contribute to placental transfusion and are outlined in the comment section of **Table 1**. In normal full-term newborn infants, the increase in blood volume has been estimated to be 33% at 30 minutes and 17% at 4 hours of age, at which time it stabilizes because of a shift of fluid between the intra- and extravascular compartments. Earlier investigators studied placental transfusion primarily by tagging albumin and red blood cells with radioisotopes to understand whether hypervolemia and congestive heart failure had a role in the etiology of hyaline membrane disease. During the last decade, there has been a resurgence of interest in assessing the possible advantages of placental transfusion in premature infants, such as reducing the number of blood transfusions,[11–16] improving blood pressure,[16,17] decreasing intraventricular hemorrhage,[14,18,19] reducing late onset sepsis, and improving the infant's immune status due to the transfusion of hematopoietic progenitor cells.[20] Rarely, adverse effects are observed with excess placental transfusion, including polycythemia (hyperviscosity), hyperbilirubinemia, and respiratory distress due to hypervolemia.[1,21,22] A delay in clamping the cord can also slow down the initiation of resuscitation. Several reviews in recent years have documented various clinical benefits of placental transfusion in term[12] and preterm infants[11,12] and have suggested a delay in clamping the cord to facilitate placental transfusion.[1,20–22] Although extensive research has been conducted on placental transfusion, there is paucity of information on its benefits and risks in infants born by cesarean section, particularly in extremely premature infants.[14–16,20,23–27] This article reviews factors contributing to placental transfusion in infants born by cesarean section and its effects on their clinical outcome.

MEASURING PLACENTAL TRANSFUSION

The method of estimating the volume of placental transfusion may impact the results and should be considered when comparing various studies. Placental transfusion is determined by measuring neonatal blood volume, placental blood volume, or both. Plasma volume is measured by using an indicator that binds to the serum albumin, such as I^{125}, I^{131}, or Evans blue dye.[1] These indicators disappear from the circulation at the rate of 20% an hour in normal neonates and more rapidly in infants with sepsis, hypervolemia, or acidosis.[1] This decay curve may result in underestimating blood volume in newborn infants.[1] Radioisotope labeling of red blood cells has also been used to estimate red cell volume but can overestimate blood volume because of a delay in mixing time.[28] Several investigators have measured the hematocrit to assess blood volume. Although this technique is simple, it can be erroneous due to the plasma volume shift, and the methods used are often not standardized for neonatal red cells.[28,29] Recently, autologous biotinylated red blood cells have been used to measure red cell volume.[23–25] This technique not only avoids exposure to radioactive isotope but has been shown to be superior to blood volume estimate based on hematocrit.[28] Placental blood volume is measured either by simple drainage or by determination of the fetal hemoglobin content in the maternal, placental, or neonatal blood.[1,3–7,10] The simple drainage method can underestimate the placental blood volume by approximately 9 mL/kg.[1]

PLACENTAL TRANSFUSION AND BLOOD VOLUME

Several studies have evaluated the clinical conditions and factors affecting placental transfusion in infants born by cesarean section with early and late clamping of the umbilical cord (**Table 1**). These factors include the timing of cord clamping,[1,2,11–13,17] gravity,[13] the onset of respiration,[9,10] uterine contraction[30–32] and drugs affecting uterine contraction,[1,5] maternal blood pressure,[2] and birth asphyxia.[6,7] Blood volume in infants changes considerably over the first few hours of life following placental transfusion. The initial increase in blood volume stabilizes over several hours by rapid transudation of plasma.[1,3,11–13] Yao and colleagues[3] concluded that the volume of blood distributed between the term infant and the placenta was 66% and 34%, respectively. A stepwise increase in the transfer of blood between the placenta and the infant occurs from birth up to the first 3 minutes, with an estimated volume distribution of 87% and 13%, respectively.[3] The red cell volume usually stabilizes at 4 hours of age and increases by approximately 50% in full-term infants and 47% in large preterm infants. The elevated total blood volume measured with the I^{125} dilution technique at 4 hours is less pronounced when compared with the red cell volume. The estimated increase in the total blood volume in newborn infants born vaginally after 5 minutes of delay in cord clamping is 14% and 17% for term and preterm infants, respectively. A similar initial blood volume distribution is observed in infants born via cesarean section.[8,9] Strauss and colleagues[23] found an increase in the blood volume (measured by biotinylated red blood cells) in larger premature infants at 30 to 36 weeks' gestation born by vaginal delivery but not in those delivered by cesarean section. Aladangady and colleagues[25] also measured the blood volume of premature infants born by cesarean section or vaginal delivery using biotinylated autologous red blood cell. They concluded that although placental transfusion occurs with delayed cord clamping in both vaginal delivery and cesarean section, the blood volume transferred in infants born by cesarean section was not statistically significant.

Time of Cord Clamping

In healthy term newborn infants, postnatal transfer of blood from the placenta to the fetus occurs during the first 3 minutes after birth if the infant is kept at or below the placenta. The total blood volume increases by 10% to 30%; red cell mass increases by 25% to 60% as a result of late cord clamping while the plasma volume remains constant or decreases. Theoretically, plasma volume, red cell mass, and blood volume should increase proportionally during placental transfusion; however, hypervolemia and hypovolemia at the time of cord clamping are rapidly counteracted by fluid shifts to or from the extravascular space, causing increased or decreased hematocrits. Only the red cell mass remains stable during the first hours of life, and it is closely related to the blood volume at the time of cord clamping unless interference from hemolysis or bleeding occurs.[1] Because placental transfusion occurs in a stepwise manner, it is related to the time of uterine contractions. Closure of the umbilical arteries begins within 15 seconds of birth, with functional closure by 45 seconds. Closure of the umbilical vein begins by 15 seconds with the diameter decreasing significantly by 1 to 2 minutes. The blood volume of infants born by cesarean section increases when the cord is clamped at 40 seconds (see **Table 1**) but decreases thereafter.[2]

Position of the Infant

The rate of placental transfusion is influenced by the position of the infant in relation to the placenta at delivery. Infants kept 50 to 60 cm above the placenta during vaginal delivery do not receive any placental transfusion within 3 minutes of birth. Infants kept at 40 or 20 cm above the placenta receive some blood from the placenta.[1] At 10 cm above or 10 cm below the placenta, infants receive the full amount of blood within 3 minutes. Keeping the infant 40 cm below the placenta hastens placental transfusion to almost completion at about 30 seconds. The pressure generated by uterine contractions is nullified if the infant is held above the placenta at or above 50 cm during

Table 1
Placental transfusion with early versus delayed cord clamping in infants born by cesarean section

		Early Cord Clamping							Delayed Cord Clamping						
Study	Method	No.	Time	GA Week	BV (mL/kg)	RCV	PBV	No.	Time	GA Week	BV (mL/kg)	RCV (mL)	PBV (mL)	Comments
Yao[6]	I[135] albumin	13	Before birth	Term	66	—	—	—	—	—	—	—	—	Non-asphyxiated infants born by cesarean section for maternal reasons
Yao[6]	I[135] albumin	5	Before birth	Term	90	—	—	—	—	—	—	—	—	Asphyxiated infants born by cesarean section for fetal distress had increased volume compared with non-asphyxiated infants, suggesting in utero PT
Sisson[8]	Dye dilution method	8	Soon after birth	Term	87	37	—	7	3 m	Term	106	45	—	DCC results in moderate placental transfusion if infant held below the level of uterus, and reduced BV if held above ECC does not alter the blood volume compared with fetal blood volume of infants held above the uterus
Klebe[24]	Simple drainage	10	<20 s	34–41	—	—	61	3	3 m	36–39	—	—	24	Nondiabetic mothers, mostly elective cesarean section
Klebe[24]	Simple drainage	29	<20 s	32–36	—	—	77	8	3 m	35–38	—	—	42	Diabetic mothers with elective cesarean section With ECC, higher neonatal BV and lower PBV in infants born vaginally With DCC, amount of PT is similar in cesarean section and vaginal deliveries

Ogata[2]	Fetal hemoglobin level	7	Soon after birth	—	Term	—	55	13	20 s	Term	—	30	Elective cesarean section for previous cesarean section Anesthesia: 19 epidural, 1 general PT occurs in the first 40 s, then the process reverses PBV had inverse correlation with maternal blood pressure with ECC
Philip[9]	Simple drainage	—	—	—	—	—	—	13	40 s	Term	—	108	Elective cesarean section, above the level of placenta, cord clamped after infant initiation of breathing
Philip[9]	Simple drainage	—	—	—	—	—	—	16	51 s	Term	—	70	Elective cesarean section, infant below level of placenta, cord clamped after initiation of breathing Demonstrated the effect of gravity and respiration on the PT
Strauss[23]	Biotinylated RBC	10	<15 s	30–36	37	—	5	—	1 m	30–35	37	—	RCT, infant kept at the level of the uterus No significant PT with cesarean section
Aladangy[25]	Biotinylated RBC	12	—	24–32	64	—	14	—	30–90 s	24–32	70	—	RCT, PT does occur with cesarean section, difference is not statistically significant

Abbreviations: BV, blood volume; DCC, delayed cord clamping; ECC, early cord clamping; GA, gestational age; PBV, placental blood volume; PT, placental transfusion; RBC, red blood cells; RCT, randomized control trial; RCV, red cell volume.

vaginal delivery. Similar events may occur during cesarean section, although there are no data to support it. Some investigators have suggested that the infant should be placed between the mother's thighs in cesarean section deliveries before the cord is clamped. Yao and Sisson observed that, with delayed cord clamping, the amount of blood transferred depends on the position of the infant in relation to the placenta.[4,8] Infants born by cesarean section held 15 cm below the introitus had increased blood volume, whereas infants held above the level of the uterus had lower blood volume.

Onset of Respiration

The expansion of the pulmonary vascular bed after the onset of respiration may facilitate placental transfusion. This effect was first described in infants born via cesarean section by Redmond and colleagues and subsequently confirmed by Phillip and Teng.[9,10] Even when the infant was held above the level of the placenta, placental transfusion occurred in infants with established respiration.[9] In one study, infants whose umbilical cords were clamped early breathed sooner after birth than infants in whom cord clamping was delayed, and this difference was speculated to be due to the anoxia stimulating the respiration in the early clamped group.[1] Excessive placental transfusion due to delayed cord clamping may result in hypervolemia, polycythemia, possible cardiac overloading, or persistent pulmonary hypertension, leading to tachypnea in full-term infants and in infants with twin-to-twin transfusion.

Uterine Contraction and Maternal Hypotension

Oxytocin given at the onset of the third stage of labor augments placental transfusion.[5] In the absence of uterine contraction, if cord clamping is delayed, placental transfusion occurs if the infant is in the dependent position.[2] Maternal hypotension and its adverse effects on placental transfusion should be also considered in infants delivered via cesarean section.[1,3] Ogata and colleagues[2] observed that the residual placental blood volume correlated inversely with maternal blood pressure during the first 20 to 40 seconds. They observed that placental transfusion occurs in the first 20 seconds in infants born by cesarean section. They also determined that the flow reverses when the cord is clamped beyond 40 seconds. In fetal lambs, Kitterman and colleagues[30] observed a direct relationship between hypotension induced in the ewes and hypovolemia in fetal lambs.

Birth Asphyxia

Yao and Lind[6] were the first group of investigators to measure the blood volume in 5 asphyxiated and 13 non-asphyxiated term infants born by cesarean section in which the mothers received general anesthesia. The umbilical cord was cut just before the delivery of the infant to eliminate the effect of uterine contraction on placental transfusion. Blood volume was determined by labeled I^{125} albumin. In non-asphyxiated infants born by cesarean section, the blood volume after early cord clamping was similar to that in infants born by vaginal delivery (ie, 66 mL/kg), which represented fetal blood volume. Asphyxiated infants with early cord clamping had a higher blood volume of 90 mL/kg, similar to infants with delayed cord clamping. They speculated that the blood volume in asphyxiated infants increased due to in utero compensatory mechanisms in the fetus leading to increased umbilical flow. Similar observations were made by Linderkamp.[1] Kitterman and colleagues[30] studied the effect of intrauterine asphyxia on blood volume in 11 fetal lambs. They measured the fetoplacental red blood cell volume with Cr^{51} tagged red cells and plasma volume with I^{125} tagged albumin and concluded that asphyxia in lambs does not affect blood volume in fetal lambs. Data controlling for compounding factors in prematurely born asphyxiated infants delivered by cesarean section are unavailable.

PLACENTAL TRANSFUSION AND CLINICAL OUTCOME OF INFANTS BORN BY CESAREAN SECTION

The clinical outcomes of delayed cord clamping in infants born by cesarean section are summarized in **Table 2**.

Placental Transfusion in Full-Term Infants Born by Cesarean Section

Erkkola and colleagues[32] evaluated the effects of general anesthesia in term infants born by elective cesarean section in 19 healthy mothers. Thiopentone and succinylcholine were used in all of the patients without any premedication. Patients were assigned to three groups. In group 1 infants, the umbilical cord was clamped soon after birth; in group 2, it was clamped at 1.5 minutes; and in group 3, it was clamped at 3 minutes, with the groups 2 and 3 infants kept at the level of uterus. The heart rate, respiratory rate, blood pressure, hemoglobin, hematocrit, lactate, and bilirubin levels were recorded serially. Apgar scores were similar in all three groups. Respiratory acidosis developed in the infants with delayed cord clamping, and increased plasma lactate was also noted in group 3. The infants with delayed cord clamping were initially vigorous but later noted to be sleepy and comfortable. No significant clinical deterioration occurred despite the changes in the cord blood gas values. Erkkola and coworkers concluded that healthy mature infants did not benefit from delayed cord clamping following cesarean section. They speculated that the infants with delayed clamping of the cord received transplacental general anesthetic.[32] A recent review noted higher hemoglobin and hematocrit levels in term infants at 6 hours of age, higher blood volume at 24 to 48 hours of age, and an increase in ferritin levels at 3 months with a low risk of iron deficiency anemia at 6 months of age.[12] Nevertheless, only one study included infants born by cesarean section. Because the outcome of infants was not stratified by mode of delivery, and when controlling for variables contributing to placental transfusion, no conclusion can be drawn regarding the risks and benefits of delayed cord clamping in infants born by cesarean section.

Placental Transfusion in Premature Infants Born by Cesarean Section

Several investigators have documented the clinical benefits of placental transfusion in premature infants; however, most of these infants were born by vaginal delivery.[13–20,26] Several review articles have also documented the advantages of delayed cord clamping in premature infants.[11–13] In a meta-analysis of the published data, Rabe and colleagues[11,13] concluded that the benefits of placental transfusion were a greater circulating blood volume during the first day of life, a reduced need for blood transfusions, and a decrease in intraventricular hemorrhage. These studies included premature infants born by vaginal and cesarean section deliveries. Rabe and colleagues[15] concluded that delayed cord clamping up to 45 seconds is feasible and safe in premature infants less than 33 weeks' gestation delivered by cesarean section. In this study, 20 infants were born by cesarean section in the early clamped group and 15 in the delayed clamped group. A significant reduction in the need for packed red blood cell transfusion was observed at 6 weeks in the group with a delay in cord clamping, with no increase in the incidence of hyperviscosity or hyperbilirubinemia in either group.[15] Nelle and colleagues[17] studied the effects of early versus late clamping on systemic circulation and cerebral blood flow velocity in premature infants born by cesarean section.

Table 2
Effects of delayed clamping on clinical parameters in infants born by spontaneous vaginal delivery or cesarean section

Parameter	Mercer[15]		Rabe[15]		Mercer[20]		Kugelman[26]		Nelle[17]	
	Early	Delayed	Early	Delayed	Early	Delayed	Early	Delayed	Early	Delayed
Cord clamping										
No. of CS/vag	6/10	9/6	19/1	15/4	14/22	15/11	11	14	8	11
Definition	<10 s	30–45 s	20 s	45 s	<10 s	30–45 s	—	—	—	30 s
Gestation (weeks)	27 ± 2.2	28 ± 2	29	30 ± 1.57	24–31	24–31	—	—	29	30
Apgar score	6/7	6/7	8	9	7/8	7/8	—	—	—	—
Hct, initial	42 ± 9.8	44 ± 10.8	—	—	46	49	51	52	—	—
Hct, 4 h	—	—	—	—	—	—	—	—	0.46	0.55
MBP (mm of Hg), initial	30 ± 4.6	35 ± 7	—	—	—	—	36	44	—	—
MBP (mm of Hg), 4 h	30.7 ± 3.8	33.2 ± 4.3	38	38	32	34	—	—	36	44
No. with RDS	—	—	4	3	—	—	—	—	—	—
MV (mL)	16+16	13+17	8	9	—	—	—	—	—	—
No. with IVH	5	3	3	1	13	5	—	—	—	—
No. with PDA	—	—	2	2	—	—	—	—	—	—
No. with suspected NEC	14	8	—	—	20	14	—	—	—	—
BPD (%)	56	31	—	—	25	22	—	—	—	—
Volume in 24 h	—	—	7	4	—	—	—	—	—	—
No. with phototherapy	—	—	12	12	33	27	—	—	—	—
Volume transfused (mL)	62+46	40+44	—	—	—	—	—	—	—	—
Days on O2	51+41	31+36	—	—	—	—	—	—	—	—
No. discharged on O2	7	1	—	—	9	0	—	—	—	—
No. with sepsis	—	—	—	—	—	—	—	—	—	—

Abbreviations: +, increase; BPD, bronchopulmonary dysplasia; CS, cesarean section; DCC, delayed cord clamping; ECC, early cord clamping; Hct, hematocrit; IVH, intraventricular hemorrhage; MBP, mean blood pressure; MV, minute ventilation; NEC, necrotizing enterocolitis; PDA, patent ductus arteriosus; RDS, respiratory distress syndrome; Vag, vaginal delivery.

Delayed clamping was defined as 30 seconds, and all infants were kept below the level of the placenta. They concluded that delayed cord clamping increased mean blood pressure, systemic vascular resistance, hemoglobin, and systemic and cerebral hemoglobin transport in premature infants. In contrast, the group of infants with early cord clamping required more therapy with volume expanders (early, 7/8 versus late, 2/11; $P<.03$).

SUMMARY

Delayed cord clamping in infants born by cesarean section results in placental transfusion in term and premature infants. A moderate delay in cord clamping up to 30 to 40 seconds is feasible and should be practiced. Term infants may have a higher hematocrit initially and a decreased incidence of iron deficiency anemia at 6 months of age. In premature infants, several small studies have suggested that there is also a higher blood volume and hematocrit initially with a decreased incidence of intraventricular hemorrhage. The effect of compounding factors such as maternal blood pressure, uterine contraction, medications, and bleeding, and their effects on the infant's immediate and long-term outcome are unclear. The short- and long-term benefits and risks of placental transfusion in extremely low birth weight infants born by cesarean section have not been studied; therefore, multicenter trials may be warranted.

REFERENCES

1. Linderkamp O. Placental transfusion: determinants and effects. Clin Perinatol 1982;9:559–92.
2. Ogata ES, Kitterman JA, Kleinberg F, et al. The effect of time of cord clamping and maternal blood pressure on placental transfusion with cesarean section. Am J Obstet Gynecol 1977;128:197–200.
3. Yao AC, Moinian M, Lind J. Distribution of blood between the infant and the placenta after birth. Lancet 1969;7626(2):871–3.
4. Yao AC, Lind J. Effect of gravity on placental transfusion. Lancet 1969;2:505–8.
5. Yao AC, Hirvensalo M, Lind J. Placental transfusion rate and uterine contraction. Lancet 1968;1:380–3.
6. Yao AC, Lind J. Blood volume in the asphyxiated term neonate. Biol Neonate 1972;21:199–209.
7. Yao AC, Wist A, Lind T. The blood volume of the newborn infant delivered by caesarean section. Acta Paediatr Scand 1967;56:585–92.
8. Sisson TRC, Knutson S, Kendall N. The blood volume of infants. IV. Infants born by cesarean section. Am J Obstet Gynecol 1973;117:351–7.
9. Philip AGS, Teng SS. Role of respiration in effecting transfusion at cesarean section. Biol Neonate 1977;31:219–44.
10. Redmond D, Isana S, Ingal D. Relation of onset of respiration to placental transfusion. Lancet 1965;1:283–5.
11. Rabe H, Reynolds G, Diaz-Rossello J. Early versus delayed umbilical cord clamping in preterm infants. Cochrane Database Syst Rev 2004;(4):CD003248.
12. Hutton EK, Hassan SE. Late vs. early clamping of the umbilical cord in full-term neonates: systematic review and meta-analysis of controlled trials. JAMA 2007; 297:1241–52.
13. Rabe H, Reynolds G, Diaz-Rossello J. A systematic review and meta-analysis of a brief delay in clamping the umbilical cord of preterm infants. Neonatology 2008; 93:138–44.

14. Mercer JS, McGrath MM, Hensman A, et al. Immediate and delayed cord clamping in infants born between 24 and 32 weeks: a pilot randomized controlled trial. J Perinatol 2003;23:466–72.

15. Rabe H, Wacker A, Hülskamp G, et al. A randomized controlled trial of delayed cord clamping in very low birth weight preterm infants. Eur J Pediatr 2000;159: 775–7.

16. Ibrahim HM, Krouskop RW, Lewis DF, et al. Placental transfusion: umbilical cord clamping and preterm infants. J Perinatol 2000;20:351–4.

17. Nelle M, Fisher S, Conze S, et al. Effects of late cord clamping on circulation in prematures. Pediatr Res 1998;44:454.

18. Hofmeyr GJ, Bolton KD, Bowen DC, et al. Periventricular/intraventricular hemorrhage and umbilical cord clamping. S Afr Med J 1988;73:104–6.

19. Hofmeyer GJ, Gobetz L, Bex PJ, et al. Periventricular/intraventricular hemorrhage following early and delayed umbilical cord clamping: a randomized trial. Online J Curr Clin Trials 1993;Doc No 110.

20. Mercer JS, Vohr BR, McGrath MM, et al. Delayed cord clamping in very preterm infants reduces the incidence of intraventricular hemorrhages and late-onset sepsis: a randomized, controlled trial. Pediatrics 2006;117:1235–42.

21. Peltonen T. Placental transfusion: advantage and disadvantage. Eur J Pediatr 1981;137:141–6.

22. Philip AGS, Saigal S. When should we clamp the umbilical cord? NeoReviews 2004;5:e142–53.

23. Strauss RG, Mock DM, Johnson K, et al. A randomized clinical trial comparing immediate versus delayed clamping of the umbilical cord in preterm infants: short-term clinical and laboratory endpoints. Transfusion 2008;48:658–65.

24. Klebe JG, Ingomar CJ. The influence of the method of delivery and clamping technique on the red cell volume in infants of diabetic and non-diabetic mothers. Acta Paediatr Scand 1974;63:65–9.

25. Aladangady N, McHugh S, Aitchison TC, et al. Infants' blood volume in a controlled trial of placental transfusion at preterm delivery. Pediatrics 2006;117:93–8.

26. Kugelman A, Borenstein-Levin L Riskin A, et al. Immediate versus delayed umbilical cord clamping in premature neonates born <35 weeks: a prospective, randomized, controlled study. Am J Perinatol 2007;24:307–15.

27. Kinmond S, Aitchison TC, Holland BM, et al. Umbilical cord clamping and preterm infants: a randomized trial. BMJ 1993;306:172–5.

28. Jones JG, Holland BM, Hudson I, et al. Total circulating red cell volume versus hematocrit as the primary descriptor of oxygen transport by the blood. Br J Haematol 1990;76:288–94.

29. Villalta JA, Pramanik AK, Diaz BJ, et al. Diagnostic error in neonatal polycythemia based on the method of hemocrit determination. J Pediatr 1989;115:460–2.

30. Kitterman JA, Schlueter, Phibbs RH. Effects of intrauterine asphyxia on neonatal blood volume. Pediatr Res 1974;8:447.

31. Pramanik AK. Impact on the newborn: physiological consequences of being born by cesarean. In: Alfonso DA, editor. Impact of cesarean childbirth. 1st edition. Philadelphia: FA Davis; 1981. p. 113–29.

32. Erkkola R, Kero P, Kanto J, et al. Delayed cord clamping in cesarean section with general anesthesia. Am J Perinatol 1984;1:165–9.

Cesarean Delivery in the Developing World

Blair J. Wylie, MD, MPH[a,b,]*, Fadi G. Mirza, MD[c]

KEYWORDS

- Cesarean delivery • International maternal health
- Health care access

The prevalence of cesarean delivery (CD) in the United States is at a record high of 31.1% of all births (2006 data), representing an increase of 50% in the past decade alone.[1] The overall rate reflects a marked upswing in the frequency of primary CD and a sharp decline in the frequency of vaginal birth after CD. In certain emerging economies, such as Brazil, CD rates are even higher, exceeding 75% in the urban private sector.[2] Practitioners and policymakers currently are struggling to clarify whether these high rates are acceptable. Increasing maternal requests for primary CD and societal and litigious pressures to avoid all birth-related injuries are being balanced against the known complications of surgery, the associated increased costs, and the impact on future pregnancies.

At a time when developed nations are beginning to examine critically this continued increase in surgical deliveries, women in many parts of the world do not even have access to the procedure. Approximately 12% of deliveries are estimated to occur via CD in the developing world—as low as 8% if births in China are excluded.[3] In many of these countries, particularly among the rural and the poor populations, the proportion of births delivered by cesarean is drastically lower. The World Health Organization (WHO) advocates an "optimal" national CD rate between 5% and 15% of all births, which suggests that levels less than 5% indicate limited availability for a significant proportion of the population.[4] This article reviews CD rates in the least developed countries compared with rates in countries with advanced or emerging economies. Barriers to access are highlighted, and the impact on maternal and perinatal mortality and morbidity is evaluated. The trend leading to excessively high CD rates in countries with emerging economies, such as Brazil and China, also are examined.

---

[a] Harvard Medical School, Division of Maternal-Fetal Medicine, Department of Obstetrics and Gynecology, Massachusetts General Hospital, 55 Fruit Street, Boston, MA 02115, USA
[b] Center for International Health and Development, Boston University School of Public Health, Boston, MA, USA
[c] Division of Maternal-Fetal Medicine, Department of Obstetrics and Gynecology, Columbia University, 622 West 168th Street, PH 16-66, New York, NY 10032, USA
* Corresponding author. Department of Obstetrics and Gynecology, Massachusetts General Hospital, 55 Fruit Street, Boston, MA 02115.
E-mail address: bwylie@partners.org (B.J. Wylie).

Clin Perinatol 35 (2008) 571–582
doi:10.1016/j.clp.2008.06.002
0095-5108/08/$ – see front matter © 2008 Elsevier Inc. All rights reserved.

perinatology.theclinics.com

BACKGROUND

The label "developing country" is often inappropriately attached to any country that is not fully developed. The term implies that economic development and progress are occurring, yet many poor countries have experienced ongoing economic decline. On the other hand, some developing countries have demonstrated impressive economic growth and increasing industrialization (eg, Brazil, China, Egypt, India, Mexico, Poland, Russia, South Africa, South Korea, and Turkey).[5] Lumping these types of countries under one designation—developing country—incorrectly suggests comparable standards of living, economic situations, and access to health care. The International Monetary Fund divides the world into two groups: (1) advanced economies and (2) emerging and developing countries.[6] Among the latter group, the United Nations (UN) further designates 33 African, 15 Asian, and 1 Caribbean nation as the least developed nations (**Fig. 1**).[7] For purposes of this article, we attempt to distinguish, when possible, among nations with advanced economies, nations with emerging markets, and nations that are the least developed to highlight distinct trends.

PREVALENCE

A major obstacle to determining accurate estimates of CD rates in developing countries is the lack of reliable data at the national level.[8] Vital statistics registries, when they do exist, may not capture the mode of delivery. Population-based CD rates are primarily derived from demographic and health surveys, which are highly standardized surveys of nationally representative samples of women of reproductive age. Questions regarding obstetric care, including method of delivery, are asked of any woman who reported a live birth in the 3 to 5 years before the survey. Interviewers are trained to clarify that CD is defined as delivery through an abdominal incision so as to not confuse it with operative vaginal deliveries or episiotomies. To calculate the rate, the number of self-reported CDs is divided by the number of live births among interviewees in the same time period. Despite their widespread use, the accuracy of

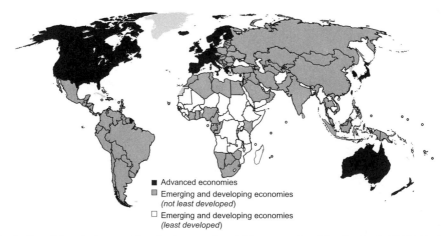

■ Advanced economies
▨ Emerging and developing economies
(not least developed)
☐ Emerging and developing economies
(least developed)

Fig. 1. Countries designated by the International Monetary Fund in the April 2008 World Economic Outlook as advanced economies are shown in black, whereas countries designated as emerging and developing countries are in gray and white, the latter color representing countries designated by the United Nations as least developed countries.

the data generated by this approach has not been validated.[8] In addition to the demographic and health surveys, data on national CD rates are extrapolated from facility-based studies that rely on review of institutional records to determine the number of CDs performed in a given region. CD rates are then calculated for that region by dividing the CD number by the number of live births reported in the region served by that facility.

Acknowledging limitations in data accuracy, Stanton and Holtz[3] estimated CD rates for 82 individual countries. Their primary source of the information was the demographic health surveys described previously. The reference period was between 1996 and 2003 and, when available, comparisons were made with rates estimated from 1986 to 1994 data. During this time period, 1 in 12 births in the developing world was performed via CD. Notably, marked global variation was evident with regional rates as follows: East Asia (26.3%), West Asia (11.9%), South Asia (7.5%), Southeast Asia (4.6%), Eurasia (5.4%), Latin America/Caribbean (25.8%), North Africa (9.5%), and Sub-Saharan Africa (2.9%). Country-specific rates are presented in **Table 1**, with least developed nations shaded in gray. Comparable regional rates were estimated by Betrán and colleagues[9] using data from additional sources when nationally representative surveys or vital statistics were not available.

What is evident from the figures reported by Stanton and Holtz and Betrán and colleagues is the drastic difference in CD rates between the least developed nations and the remaining developing world. **Fig. 2** displays the regional CD rates presented by Stanton divided into three groups according to the WHO definition of the "optimal" rate: (1) less than 5%, (2) 5% to 15% (optimal), and (3) more than 15%.[4] Twenty-three of the 25 least developed countries (92%) had CD rates lower than 5% of all births compared with only 11 of the 57 more advanced/emerging economies (19%).[3] In the study by Betrán and colleagues,[9] a similar disparity was demonstrated. The CD rate was estimated at 21.1% for developed regions of the world, 14.3% among less developed countries, and 2% for the least developed countries.

Variability in CD rates also seems to differ markedly within countries and between them. In the study by Stanton and Holtz,[3] urban rates were approximately three times higher than rural CD rates in the 36 countries sampled with available data (**Table 1**). Variations in method of delivery between urban and rural populations were noted in another analysis of 42 developing nations.[10] These researchers reported rates by wealth quintile and by urban versus rural residence. Rates were remarkably low among the poorest women. Less than 1% of women in the poorest quintile in roughly half of the studied nations had CD. In the remaining half, CD rates for the poorest quintile did not achieve the minimum WHO standard of 5%, with only a few exceptions noted. When plotted as CD rates by urban versus rural rich versus rural poor, the differences are striking (**Fig. 3**). At the other extreme, the CD rate for the richest quintile exceeded the 2006 US rate in 20% of the countries examined. In the Dominican Republic and Brazil, for example, rates for the richest women surpassed 50% (54.5% and 67.6%, respectively).

From the available data, two trends are apparent regarding CD in the developing world. In the least developed countries and even for rural women and poor women in the emerging economies, access to the procedure remains limited, which raises questions of safety for mother and fetus. Perhaps equally disturbing is the dramatic increase in CD in other regions, most notably in parts of Latin America and Asia. Safety concerns are equally valid when more than half of women in certain socioeconomic groups are undergoing CD. The optimal minimum and maximum CD rates continue to be a matter of debate and may never be resolved.[11–13] The two extremes evident in the developing world deserve critical examination.

Table 1
Cesarean delivery rate by country

Region/Country	CD Rate (Overall) %	CD Rate (Urban) %	CD Rate (Rural) %
North Africa			
Algeria	4.9	—	—
Egypt	11.4	18.2	7.1
Libya	7.2	—	—
Morocco	5.4	—	—
Tunisia	8.0	—	—
Sub-Saharan Africa			
Benin	3.5	7.7	1.6
Burkina Faso	0.7	2.8	0.3
Cameroon	2.5	3.4	2.1
Central African Republic	1.9	—	—
Chad	0.4	—	—
Comoros	5.3	—	—
Côte d'Ivoire	2.5	4.9	1.4
Eritrea	1.6	—	—
Ethiopia	0.6	—	—
Gabon	6.0	—	—
Ghana	3.7	7.6	1.8
Kenya	4.0	9.4	2.8
Madagascar	0.6	—	—
Malawi	2.7	4.4	2.4
Mali	1.2	3.5	0.5
Mauritania	3.3	5.6	1.5
Mozambique	2.7	—	—
Namibia	6.9	—	—
Niger	0.6	2.1	0.3
Nigeria	1.7	3.5	1.0
Rwanda	2.3	7.2	1.4
Senegal	5.0	6.0	4.3
South Africa	15.4	—	—
Sudan	3.7	—	—
Tanzania	3.0	6.5	2.1
Togo	2.0	—	—
Uganda	2.6	8.0	1.9
Zambia	2.2	4.4	1.2
Zimbabwe	7.4	10.2	6.0
Latin America/Caribbean			
Argentina	25.4	—	—
Bolivia	14.7	31.4	6.0
Brazil	36.7	—	—
Chile	40.0	—	—
Colombia	25.2	30.3	14.1

(continued on next page)

Table 1
(continued)

Region/Country	CD Rate (Overall) %	CD Rate (Urban) %	CD Rate (Rural) %
Costa Rica	20.8	—	—
Cuba	23.0	—	—
Dominican Republic	31.3	34.7	24.9
Ecuador	19.9	27.6	10.7
El Salvador	15.7	21.4	—
Guatemala	11.7	20.8	6.0
Haiti	1.7	3.3	0.9
Honduras	9.6	12.9	4.7
Mexico	24.1	—	—
Nicaragua	14.7	22.4	7.1
Panama	18.2	—	—
Paraguay	16.5	31.5	6.2
Peru	12.9	21.0	3.2
Uruguay	21.9	—	—
Venezuela	21.0	—	—
East Asia			
China	25.9	—	—
South Korea	37.7	—	—
South Asia			
Bangladesh	2.7	—	—
India	7.1	14.7	4.9
Iran	29.8	—	—
Nepal	1.0	5.0	0.7
Pakistan	2.9	—	—
Southeast Asia			
Cambodia	1.0	—	—
Indonesia	4.1	6.6	1.9
Philippines	7.3	9.8	4.7
Vietnam	3.4	—	—
West Asia			
Bahrain	16.0	—	—
Jordan	16.0	16.3	14.8
Kuwait	11.2	—	—
Lebanon	15.1	—	—
Oman	6.6	—	—
Palestine	6.1	—	—
Qatar	15.9	—	—
Saudi Arabia	8.1	—	—
Syria	14.8	—	—
Turkey	17.1	21.5	10.0
United Arab Emirates	9.6	—	—
Yemen	1.5	—	—

(continued on next page)

Table 1 (continued)			
Region/Country	CD Rate (Overall) %	CD Rate (Urban) %	CD Rate (Rural) %
Eurasia			
Armenia	7.4	—	—
Kazakhstan	10.8	15.2	7.7
Kyrgyz Republic	6.0	—	—
Turkmenistan	3.6	—	—
Uzbekistan	3.0	—	—

Countries shaded in gray represent least developed countries according to United Nations designation.

Abbreviation: —, not available.

Data from Stanton CK, Holtz SA. Levels and trends in cesarean birth in the developing world. Stud Fam Plann 2006;37(1):41–7.

LIMITED ACCESS IN LEAST DEVELOPED COUNTRIES

Obstetric practice in least developed countries is plagued by challenges that seem implausible in the developed world. For many women, there simply is no nearby facility at which CD is an option. The capability of a facility to perform CD is considered by the UN and WHO as one of the key indicators of comprehensive emergency obstetric care.[4] Over the past decade, increasing attention has been paid to the availability and distribution of comprehensive emergency obstetric care facilities in the developing world in an effort to reduce unacceptably high maternal mortality ratios. Formal needs assessments of emergency obstetric care availability have demonstrated that in hospitals providing obstetric care in select African countries, the proportion without the ability to perform CD may be more than 75%.[14] Similarly, in certain regions of India and Nepal, two thirds of surveyed hospitals providing obstetric care were not capable of performing CD. These figures do not include nonhospital health care facilities that provide obstetric care, at which CD is almost universally unavailable.

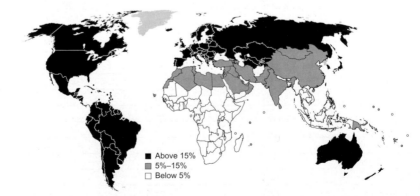

Fig. 2. CD rates by world region grouped according to designation by the United Nations. Rates are divided into three categories: less than 5% (*white*), 5% to 15% (*gray*), and more than 15% (*black*), which represent below minimal, optimal, and above maximal CD rates, respectively, as recommended by the World Health Organization.

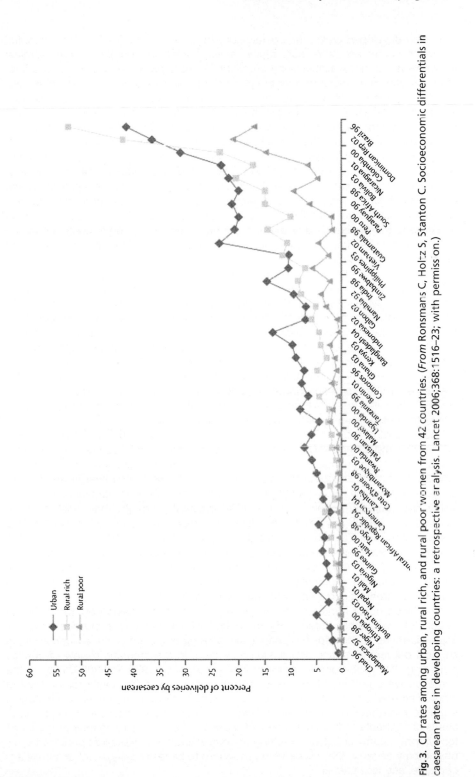

Fig. 3. CD rates among urban, rural rich, and rural poor women from 42 countries. (*From* Ronsmans C, Holz S, Stanton C. Socioeconomic differentials in caesarean rates in developing countries: a retrospective analysis. Lancet 2006;368:1516–23; with permiss on.)

In least developed areas, the obstacles to the provision of CD at a given hospital or health center are numerous. Many facilities lack an operating room, surgical instruments, or an available surgeon. Even in settings in which CD is possible, many facilities are unable to offer the procedure reliably and safely at all times secondary to gaps in provider coverage, electrical or water outages, and inconsistent supply of essential drugs and equipment.[15] There are limited or nonexistent blood banks or protocols to protect against life-threatening transfusion reactions.[16] Anesthesia services are often woefully inadequate. In a survey of anesthetists practicing in 77 hospitals in Uganda, Malawi, and Zambia, only 6% reported the ability to provide safe anesthesia for CD.[17] Electricity was only partially available in 65% of these facilities and was never available in an additional 14%. Local repair of broken equipment, such as oxygen concentrators or suction devices, is often not feasible, which translates into a reality of broken equipment remaining broken. Regional anesthesia, the preferred safer method during pregnancy, is underused secondary to inadequate training of providers, lack of appropriate spinal needles, and shortage of local anesthetic drugs.[18]

Other barriers to CD access are driven by the general level of poverty and underdevelopment. Distances to a facility that provides surgical delivery may be prohibitive for many women living in remote—particularly rural—areas. Even in more densely populated areas, the geographic distribution of comprehensive emergency obstetric care facilities may be inequitable, with poorer populations remaining underserved. Transportation may be impossible at certain times of the year secondary to impassable roads (eg, rainy season), and transport may not be accomplished in the timeframe needed to prevent injury or death to the mother or fetus or both. The cost of CD may be exorbitant for many women and serve as an additional deterrent to care. In an illustrative analysis in Madagascar, the price of a CD was, on average, 1.5 times higher than the average monthly income for these families.[19]

Nearly 100% of maternal deaths occur in the developing world.[20] The obvious question is what impact limited CD access has on maternal and fetal survival. A map of regional maternal mortality ratios categorized as high, medium, or low would look virtually identical to **Fig. 2**. An association between CD rates and maternal and neonatal survival has been demonstrated. In 59 low-income countries evaluated in one study, the neonatal mortality rate per 1000 live births was inversely related to the CD rate ($r = -0.78$, $P < .001$).[21] Similarly, the maternal mortality ratio per 100,000 live births and the CD rate were inversely associated ($r = -0.61$, $P < .001$). As the CD rate increased, fewer mothers and infants died. Reductions in maternal and neonatal mortality with increasing CD rates were confirmed in another analysis of 126 countries representing almost 90% of live births worldwide.[9] The strength of the association was greatest in regions with high maternal and neonatal mortality.

When CDs occur in areas with limited access, they are being performed for the benefit of the mother. Intervening on behalf of the fetus to prevent stillbirth or asphyxia-related handicaps has been a luxury relegated to areas of the world in which surgical delivery is routine and presumably safe. In a systematic review of studies regarding CD in sub-Saharan Africa published between 1970 and 2000, 75% of the surgeries were performed for maternal indications, most frequently for protracted labor or hemorrhage (ie, abruption, previa).[22] Symphysiotomy, relegated to a historical footnote in textbooks in the developed world, is still considered an alternative to CD in cases of obstructed labor. In a survey of Nigerian women regarding their preferences for symphysiotomy or CD in the setting of obstructed labor, two thirds preferred symphysiotomy because they viewed the procedure to be less costly, more culturally acceptable, and less painful.[23]

As highlighted in many of the national emergency obstetric care needs assessments performed in the developing world over the last decade, many facilities that lack the ability to perform CD are unfortunately not able to offer operative vaginal delivery either.[14,15] Labors may remain obstructed for prolonged periods of time. Even if the mother survives, she may still experience significant morbidities, such as the development of vesicovaginal fistulas.

Although the optimal CD rate is likely to remain undefined, there is undeniably a huge unmet need for lifesaving obstetric surgery in many areas of the world, particularly among the rural and the poor populations in the least developed countries. With increased access to and availability of CD, women living in these areas can anticipate an increase in survival for themselves and their children. Improvements in the consistent supply of medications, equipment, and trained personnel are also required to ensure that the operation itself is not associated with unacceptable rates of sepsis, hemorrhage, and maternal death, however.

CESAREAN DELIVERY AS AN EMERGING CULTURAL NORM IN MORE ADVANCED DEVELOPING NATIONS

In contrast to the least developed nations, where rates have remained alarmingly low and unchanged, the more advanced regions of the developing world have experienced an overall increase in the proportion of CDs over the past decade, presumably reflecting an improvement in health care access.[3] The UN notes that the number of deliveries performed by a skilled attendant increased globally from 41% to 57% during the 1990s, with an increasingly higher proportion performed by physicians.[24]

Although these trends should be applauded, it is concerning that in certain segments of the developing world astonishing rates of CD have been observed. This is a well-documented phenomenon in Latin America.[8,9,25,26] In an evaluation of CD rates in Latin America, 12 of the 19 countries examined—accounting for more than 80% of the deliveries in this region—had national rates above the WHO "optimal" maximum of 15%.[25] The highest national rate was found in Chile, where 40% of all births in the country were accomplished via CD.[25,27] CD rates are significantly higher for women who delivered in private institutions, which highlights disparities in health care practice between the rich and the poor. Using data from the 2005 WHO global survey on maternal and perinatal health, the median rate of CD at private institutions in Latin America was 51%, such that women delivering at these facilities were more likely to undergo CD than vaginal delivery.[26] Similar observations have been documented by other authors[2,25], with a CD frequency rate reported as high as 77% in the richest tenth percentile of Brazilian women.[10]

Latin America is not the only region of the developing world experiencing such dramatic CD rates. South Korea has a national CD rate that approaches 40%.[3] Nationally representative data are not readily available for China; however, in a review of 11 published studies detailing more than 1.25 million births primarily in urban areas, the unweighted mean CD rate in China was 40.5%.[9] Data from southern China demonstrated an overall increase in the CD rate from 22% in 1994 to 56% in 2006, with a corresponding increase in CD on maternal request rising from 0.8% to 20% in the same time period.[28]

CD is effectively becoming the cultural norm, at least for women of means in many parts of Latin America and China.[27] The factors underlying the rising popularity of CD in these regions of the world are unclear. Body image may play a role with women under the presumption that CD protects against urinary incontinence, pelvic prolapse, and sexual dissatisfaction.[29] In China, there is little tolerance of fetal risk when only one child is permitted; CD there is perceived as safer.[30] The one-child policy also has effectively eliminated concerns about the impact of a uterine scar on subsequent pregnancies. Misconceptions undoubtedly also contribute. Some Chinese women surveyed requested CD to ensure an auspicious date of birth.[31] Others cite beliefs that babies delivered surgically are smarter, as evidenced by a better head shape.[31]

The correlation between rising CD rates and improvements in maternal and perinatal survival is less evident in these more advanced emerging economies. The study that demonstrated decrements in maternal and neonatal mortality in low-income countries as CD rates rose failed to find this association in middle- or high-income countries.[21] Similarly, in areas in which maternal and neonatal mortality is already low, increasing the proportion of babies delivered by CD does not result in further improvements in maternal or neonatal survival.[9] In an analysis of more than 100,000 births from 120 institutions in eight Latin American countries, the relationship between CD and perinatal outcomes was explored.[26] Higher CD rates were associated with several negative maternal outcomes, specifically prolonged hospitalization, increased postpartum antibiotic use, and a greater need for blood transfusion. An increase in the CD rate was also significantly associated with a higher risk for severe maternal morbidity and mortality, a higher risk for fetal death, and a higher risk for neonatal intensive care admission, even in the adjusted model. Rates of preterm delivery and neonatal mortality increased once the CD rate exceeded 10%. In a separate report, an approximate threefold increase in the odds of maternal mortality after CD was reported in the public sector in Sao Paulo (aOR 3.3, 95% CI 2.6-4.3).[2] Despite its remarkable popularity in certain emerging developing nations, CD carries significant risks, and its un-indicated use may be causing harm.

SUMMARY

CD is inextricably linked with wealth at national and individual levels. The alarmingly low rates of CD in least developed nations represent a failure on the part of the global society to care for the most vulnerable populations. Increasing access to CD for women who live in these countries will increase maternal survival, decrease maternal morbidities, and likely improve neonatal survival. Increasing access to safe CD requires more than simply building operating rooms. Significant commitments must be made to improving the geographic distribution of health facilities, training and retention of obstetric and anesthetic providers, consistent supply of medications and supplies, and affordability of the procedure. At the other extreme, in the more advanced regions of the developing world, where CD rates are exponentially rising, extreme caution is warranted. Widespread espousal of CD actually may be doing more harm than good for mothers and their infants.

REFERENCES

1. Hamilton BE, Martin JA, Ventura SJ. Births: preliminary data for 2006. National vital statistics reports. Hyattsville (MD): National Center for Health Statistics; 2007.
2. Kilsztjan S, Carmo MS, Machado LC Jr, et al. Caesarean sections and maternal mortality in Sao Paulo. Eur J Obstet Gynecol Reprod Biol 2007;132(1):64–9.
3. Stanton C, Holtz S. Levels and trends in cesarean birth in the developing world. Stud Fam Plann 2006;37(1):41–8.
4. UNICEF, WHO, UNFPA. Guidelines for monitoring the availability and use of obstetric services. Available at: http://www.alianzaipss.org/reproductive-health/publications/unicef/index.html. Accessed May 18, 2008.

5. Yale University Library. Emerging markets: the big ten countries. Available at: http://www.library.yale.edu/socsci/emerge/bigten.html. Accessed May 18, 2008.

6. World Economic Outlook Database. International monetary fund emerging and developing economies list. Available at: http://www.imf.org/external/pubs/ft/weo/2008/01/weodata/groups.htm#oem. Accessed May 18, 2008.

7. The United Nations. The least developed countries: country profiles. Available at: http://www.unohrlls.org/en/ldc/related/62/. Accessed May 18, 2008.

8. Stanton CK, Dubourg D, De Broiwere V, et al. Reliability of data on caesarean sections in developing countries. Bull World Health Organ 2005;83(6):449–55.

9. Betrán AP, Merinaldi M, Lauer JA, et al. Rates of caesarean section: analysis of global, regional and national estimates. Paediatr Perinat Epidemiol 2007;21:98–113.

10. Ronsmans C, Holtz S, Stanton C. Socioeconomic differentials in caesarean rates in developing countries: a retrospective analysis. Lancet 2006;368:1516–23.

11. Peskin EG, Reine GM. What is the correct caesarean rate and how do we get there? Obstet Gynecol Surv 2002;57:189–90.

12. Hall MF. What is the right number of caesarean sections? Lancet 1997;349(9064):1557.

13. Ash AK, Okoh D. What is the right number of caesarean sections? Lancet 1997; 349(9064):1557.

14. Bailey P, Paxton A, Lobis S, et al. The availability of life-saving obstetric services in developing countries: an in-depth look at the signal functions for emergency obstetric care. Int J Gynaecol Obstet 2006;93(3):285–91.

15. Pearson L, Shoo R. Availability and use of emergency obstetric services: Kenya, Rwanda, Southern Sudan, and Uganda. Int J Gynaecol Obstet 2005;88(2):208–15.

16. Fenton PM. Blood transfusions for caesarean section in Malawi: a study of requirements, amount given and effect on mortality. Anaesthesia 1999;54:1055–8.

17. Hodges SC, Mijumbi C, Okello M, et al. Anaesthesia services in developing countries: defining the problems. Anaesthesia 2007;62:4–11.

18. Schnittger T. Regional anesthesia in developing countries. Anaesthesia 2007; 62(Suppl 1):44–7.

19. Robitail S, Gorde S, Barrau K, et al. How much does a caesarean section cost in Madagascar? Socio-economical aspects and caesarean section rate in Toamasina, Madagascar, 1999–2001. Bull Soc Pathol Exot 2004;97(4):274–9 [Article in French].

20. WHO, UNICEF. Revised 1990 estimates of maternal mortality: a new approach by WHO and UNICEF. Pan American Journal of Public Health 1997,1(6):481–5.

21. Althabe F, Sosa C, Belizán JM, et al. Cesarean section rates and maternal and neonatal mortality in low-, medium-, and high-income countries: an ecological study. Birth 2006;33(4):270–7.

22. Dumon A, de Bernis L, Bouvier-Colle MH, et al. Caesarean section rate for maternal indication in sub-Saharan Africa: a systematic review. Lancet 2001;358:1328–33.

23. Onah HE, Ugona MC. Preferences for cesarean section or symphysiotomy for obstructed labor among Nigerian women. Int J Gynaecol Obstet 2004;84(1):79–81.

24. United Nations Statistics Division. Progress towards the Millennium Development Goals, 1990–2004. Available at: http://www.millenniumindicators.un.org/unsd/mdg/SeriesDetail.aspx?srid=570&. Accessed May 14, 2008.

25. Belizan JM, Althabe F, Barros FC, et al. Rates and implications of cesarean sections in Latin America: ecological study. BMJ 1999;319:1397–402.

26. Villar J, Valladares E, Wojdyla D, et al. Caesarean delivery rates and pregnancy outcomes: the 2005 WHO global survey on maternal and perinatal health in Latin America. Lancet 2006;367(95):1819–29.

27. de Mello E, Souza C. C-sections as ideal births: the cultural constructions of beneficence and patients' rights in Brazil. Camb Q Healthc Ethics 1994;3(3):358–66.

28. Zhang J, Liu Y, Meikle S, et al. Cesarean delivery on maternal request in southeast China. Obstet Gynecol 2008;111(5):1077–82.
29. Minkoff H, Powderly K, Chervenak F, et al. Ethical dimensions of elective primary cesarean delivery. Obstet Gynecol 2004;103:387–92.
30. Feng L, Yue Y. Analysis on the 45-year cesarean rate and its social factors. Med Soc 2002;15:14–6.
31. Yao LW. A study on social factors affecting cesarean section delivery rate. Journal of the People Liberation Army Nursing 2003;20:17–8.

Impact of Route of Delivery on Continence and Sexual Function

Kyle J. Wohlrab, MD*, Charles R. Rardin, MD

KEYWORDS

• Incontinence • Mode of delivery • Sexual function

The number of cesarean sections in the United States has increased by 50% over the past decade[1] and primary elective cesareans made up 28.3% of all cesarean sections in 2001.[2] The reason for the increase in cesarean rates is debated, but is likely a combination of physician practices and maternal requests. In 2007, The American College of Obstetricians and Gynecologists released a Committee Opinion titled "Cesarean Delivery on Maternal Request." They estimated that 2.5% of all cesarean births are caused by maternal request "in the absence of any medical or obstetric indication."[3] One of the reasons cited for the rise in requests is the fear of developing stress or fecal incontinence following a vaginal delivery. The true effect of pregnancy and route of delivery on urinary incontinence, fecal incontinence, and sexual function continues to be debated as maternal requests for primary cesarean section continue to rise. A woman has a lifetime risk of undergoing one operation for urinary incontinence of 11.1%.[4] This number is also likely to increase with the aging of the population. This article reviews the current evidence on the putative protective effects of cesarean section on pelvic floor disorders.

Physiologic changes occur during pregnancy that may have lasting effects on the maternal pelvis. During childbirth, tissue stretching and tearing, neurologic and vascular compression and compromise, and muscle strain are inevitable. The levator ani complex of the pubococcygeus, puborectalis, and iliococcygeus muscles must allow passage of the fetus. The perineal body and external anal sphincter may become injured, with or without episiotomy, but sometimes as a necessary maneuver to allow passage of the fetal head or shoulders. The traumatic insults may lead to permanent damage and subsequent urinary or anal incontinence. The degree of such injuries and the natural history of subsequent pelvic floor dysfunction are largely unknown. Much of the research done has relied on retrospective questionnaires. Although these

Division of Urogynecology, Alpert Medical School of Brown University, Division of Urogynecology, Women and Infants' Hospital of Rhode Island, 695 Eddy Street, Suite 12, Providence, RI 02903, USA
* Corresponding author.
E-mail address: kwohlrab@wihri.org (K.J. Wohlrab).

Clin Perinatol 35 (2008) 583–590
doi:10.1016/j.clp.2008.06.001   perinatology.theclinics.com
0095-5108/08/$ – see front matter © 2008 Elsevier Inc. All rights reserved.

studies are subject to recall bias and other forms of error, they provide much of what is known about the natural history and development of urinary and fecal incontinence.

The true prevalence of pelvic floor dysfunction, including urinary and fecal incontinence, is unknown and difficult to quantify. Published studies suggest ranges from 5% to 44%; the discrepancy largely is based on definitions of "dysfunction." For example, elucidating objective evidence about the type and severity of urinary incontinence through physical examinations requires far more time and resources than querying the subjective reports of incontinence from a cohort of women through questionnaires. Unfortunately, subjective reporting often overestimates rates of urinary incontinence (eg, women may report wetness caused by vaginal discharge) and proves difficult when attempting to define severity (eg, "a lot" to one woman may equal "a dribble" to another). To complicate further the goal of estimating prevalence rates of incontinence, studies aimed at identifying rates of anal incontinence must define whether they include the leakage of flatus within their definition. Throughout this article, anal incontinence refers to the leakage of stool and flatus, whereas fecal incontinence defines solely the leakage of stool, whether it is liquid or solid. Rates of anal incontinence are, by definition, higher than those of fecal incontinence alone.

THE EFFECT OF ROUTE OF DELIVERY ON URINARY INCONTINENCE

Vaginal delivery has been historically linked to development of stress urinary incontinence, the mechanisms being both mechanical and neurologic. Several studies have linked vaginal delivery to injury of the pudendal nerve.[5,6] In addition, injury to the pudendal nerve during childbirth has been associated with stress urinary incontinence.[7] Furthermore, the number of vaginal deliveries is thought to be correlated with severity of incontinence, but these conclusions are based largely on expert opinion, epidemiologic studies, and assumptions between cause and effect. With the estimated $19.5 billion spent annually on urinary incontinence in the United States,[8] there has been a push for new research into the cause of stress urinary incontinence and its association with childbirth. Large epidemiologic studies have been performed to elucidate better the link between route of delivery and the development of urinary incontinence. One of the largest epidemiologic studies was performed in Norway.[9] The authors sought to examine whether women who underwent vaginal delivery during their lifetime had a higher rate of urinary incontinence than those who delivered by cesarean section. In this study, known as the EPINCONT study, 15,307 Norwegian women were surveyed about the presence and severity of any urinary incontinence. The surveys were then linked to the Norwegian national database in which delivery information for each survey respondent had been stored since 1967. The authors found that overall, 10.1% of nulliparous women complained of urinary incontinence, 15.9% of women who delivered by cesarean section, and 21% who had only vaginal deliveries. When the authors stratified urinary incontinence by age groups, the apparent protective effect of cesarean section attenuated with increasing age. By the age of 50, urinary incontinence was seen in 28.6% of women with previous cesareans compared with 30% of women with previous vaginal delivers with similar rates of moderate to severe incontinence (14.3% versus 14.2%, respectively).

Other short-term prospective studies have confirmed the association between the development of stress urinary incontinence and vaginal delivery. Van Brummen and colleagues[10] conducted a prospective cohort study of 344 primiparous Dutch women with singleton pregnancies beginning in their second trimester. The women were assessed for urinary tract symptoms at multiple time points during their pregnancy and the first postpartum year. The authors demonstrated that stress incontinence was more prevalent in women who had a vaginal delivery. They found that 33.9% of women delivering vaginally (compared with only 7.5% of those delivered by cesarean) complained of stress incontinence. At 12 months postpartum, the numbers had increased to 40.5% and 21.7%, respectively, for each group. Although these differences were statistically significant, the rates of urinary urgency, frequency, and urge incontinence were not statistically significant between the two groups at 12 months postpartum. In contrast, the CAPS trial performed by the Pelvic Floor Disorders Network in 2006 found no statistical difference in rates of stress urinary incontinence.[11] The study recruited 921 women from 11 sites across the United States and assessed rates of stress incontinence through validated surveys at 6 weeks and 6 months postpartum. Urinary incontinence at 6 months postpartum was found to be 31.3% in women delivering vaginally and 22.9% in those delivering by cesarean. When only stress incontinence was examined, there was no difference between women delivering vaginally (14.4%) and those delivering by cesarean (14.3%). Altman and colleagues[12] surveyed 395 Swedish women 10 years after their first vaginal or cesarean delivery to assess the development of urinary symptoms. Two hundred women with a mean age of 39.9 years delivered only by vaginal delivery, whereas 195 women with a mean age of 41.5 years delivered only by cesarean. Forty percent of women delivering vaginally compared with 28% of those delivering by cesarean reported stress urinary incontinence (odds ratio [OR] 3.1), but these differences were largely caused by discrepancies reported by women complaining of mild symptoms (less than one episode per week). Women complaining of more than one episode of stress incontinence weekly were found with similar frequency in each group.

In 2005, Goldberg and colleagues[13] published a study in which they had surveyed identical twin sisters at the annual Twins Days Festival in Twinsburg, Ohio. A total of 271 pairs completed validated surveys assessing symptoms of stress urinary incontinence. The authors also collected data on previous births and mode of delivery. They found that 67.1% of women with one or more vaginal deliveries reported stress incontinence compared with 47.7% of women who delivered only by cesarean and 24% of nulliparous women. Using a regression model, the authors also found that the odds of stress incontinence increased because of parity from 2.3 for one birth to 4.3 for two or more births. Furthermore, they compared rates of stress incontinence and mode of delivery between 173 parous twin sisters. Within this cohort, women who delivered vaginally were more than twice as likely (OR 2.3) as women who delivered by cesarean to report stress incontinence.

Other studies that have examined the relationship between stress urinary incontinence later in life and previous mode of delivery have concluded similar results. Handa and colleagues[14] surveyed 1293 Maryland women undergoing elective hysterectomies with validated questionnaires. They found that 36% of all those surveyed reported stress incontinence and 35% reported urge incontinence. When mode of delivery was examined, they found that 28.7% of women who had delivered exclusively by cesarean complained of stress incontinence compared with 39.1% of women with at least one vaginal delivery. Parous women who had delivered by cesarean only were 40% less likely to report stress incontinence than those who had delivered at least one child vaginally. Women with any combination of cesarean and vaginal deliveries were just as likely to report stress incontinence as those delivering only vaginally.

Connolly and colleagues[15] completed a 2-hour in-person interview of 3205 women in the Boston area to assess association between number of pregnancies, mode of delivery, and subsequent urinary symptoms. The authors found that women having at least one vaginal delivery were significantly more likely to report moderate to severe urinary incontinence than those who had never been pregnant or who had delivered only by cesarean. The effect was most pronounced in women aged 30 to 39 years old. As seen in previous studies, after the age of 40, the effect of mode of delivery on urinary incontinence was nullified. In this sample with a mean age of 49.2 years, there was no difference in the odds of moderate to severe incontinence in women who delivered solely by cesarean compared with those who had never been pregnant.

Most of the literature suggests a protective effect of elective cesarean delivery on the development of stress urinary incontinence, at least in the short-term. Women considering elective cesarean delivery to avoid incontinence should be appropriately counseled, however, that such an approach does not eliminate their risk. Buchsbaum and colleagues[16] surveyed 149 nuns in Rochester, New York, to identify rates of stress incontinence in a cohort of nulliparous women. The mean age was 68 years old. Using questionnaires, they found that 29.7% reported symptoms consistent with stress incontinence, 24.3% complained of urge incontinence, and 35.1% of nuns reported mixed incontinence symptoms. These high rates of incontinence are similar to those found in women over the age of 60 in the EPINCONT study, suggesting that pelvic floor trauma during childbirth may be negated later in life by age, menopause, and hypoestrogenism.

McKinnie and colleagues[17] surveyed 978 women, mean age 42.7 years, in relation to symptoms of urinary incontinence. Twenty-three percent reported bothersome urinary incontinence. There was no difference in rates of urinary incontinence when stratified by mode of delivery, but pregnancy itself conferred an increased risk of urinary incontinence when compared with those women who had never been pregnant (OR 2.5). The authors concluded that cesarean section was not protective against the development of urinary incontinence.

There is additional evidence that labor itself, not just delivery, may play an important role in the development of postpartum urinary incontinence. Groutz and colleagues[18] performed a prospective cohort study of 363 primiparous Israeli women. The authors assessed symptoms of stress urinary incontinence 1 year after childbirth in women who delivered vaginally, women who underwent elective cesarean sections, and women who underwent cesarean delivery for obstructed labor. The authors found that the prevalence of stress urinary incontinence was similar in women who had vaginal deliveries and women who underwent cesarean section for obstructed labor (10.3% and 12%, respectively). Furthermore, they found that only 3.4% of women who underwent planned cesarean section complained of stress urinary incontinence during that postpartum year. Although some experts have criticized studies with short-term follow-up, Altman and colleagues[19] demonstrated in a prospective survey of 229 women that symptoms in the first-year postpartum were associated with the presence of symptoms 10 years later.

Lukacz and colleagues[20] surveyed 4103 women from the Kaiser Permenante system in Southern California. Overall rates of stress urinary incontinence were 15%. When separated by previous mode of delivery, 18% of respondents having only vaginal deliveries reported stress incontinence compared with 8% of nulliparous women and 11% of women delivering by cesarean. Furthermore, in women with labored cesarean deliveries, the rates of stress incontinence were 13% compared with 5% of those who had unlabored cesareans. Although the results were not significant, the odds ratio for the development of stress incontinence was 3.9 between women delivering vaginally and those with an unlabored cesarean. Overall, vaginal delivery increased the odds of any pelvic floor disorder compared with cesarean by 85%. The authors also pointed out that the effects of modifiable risk factors, such as obesity and smoking, were powerful predictors of the development of pelvic floor dysfunction.

To summarize the available data on mode of delivery and its association with the development of postpartum urinary incontinence, Press and colleagues[21] performed a systematic analysis. In a review of all cross-sectional studies (follow-up periods ranging from 3 months to 4 years), the risk of developing stress incontinence was reduced from 16% with vaginal delivery to 10% with cesarean section, although there was only a minimal difference when only severe symptoms were considered. The authors calculated that 15 cesareans need to be performed to prevent one woman from developing stress incontinence. Following a review of published cohort studies, the rate of stress incontinence was 22% following vaginal delivery compared with 10% following cesarean section (6.6% in women delivering by elective cesarean section) resulting in a number needed to prevent of 10.

THE EFFECT OF ROUTE OF DELIVERY ON FECAL INCONTINENCE

Studies examining the relationship of fecal incontinence to vaginal delivery report a wide range of prevalence, again depending largely on differences in definitions. The relationship between vaginal delivery, especially operative delivery complicated by perineal lacerations, has been well studied. Recent evidence has suggested that occult defects in the external anal sphincter may also be sustained after what seems to be an otherwise uncomplicated vaginal delivery.[22] In addition, age plays a role in the development of anal incontinence. Zetterstrom and colleagues[23] found that increasing maternal age at delivery is a risk factor for anal incontinence, with a 30-year-old woman bearing a risk three times higher than that of a 20-year-old woman.

The CAPS study also looked at the relationship between anal sphincter tears and postpartum fecal incontinence. The Pelvic Floor Disorders Network surveyed 407 women with clinically recognized sphincter tears during vaginal delivery and compared rates of anal and fecal incontinence in women without recognized sphincter tears during vaginal delivery with those who delivered by cesarean section. Validated questionnaires were administered at 6 weeks and 6 months postpartum. As anticipated, women with third and fourth degree perineal lacerations were 2.8 times more likely to report postpartum fecal incontinence than those delivering vaginally without a sphincter tear. At 6 weeks postpartum, 26.6% of women who had sustained a sphincter tear during delivery complained of fecal incontinence compared with 11.2% of women delivering vaginally without a sphincter laceration and 10.3% of women delivering by cesarean section. At 6 months postpartum, the rates fell to 17%, 8.2%, and 7.6%, respectively. Women who delivered vaginally and did not sustain a sphincter tear had a similar prevalence of incontinence to flatus and fecal urgency as those delivering by cesarean when queried 6 months postpartum. The Network concluded that although women delivering by cesarean have lower rates of fecal incontinence 6 months postpartum, they were not immune to these types of pelvic floor dysfunction.

Fritel and colleagues[24] surveyed 2640 middle-aged French women to determine whether obstetric risk factors could be linked to complaints of fecal incontinence. The mail survey found that the prevalence of fecal incontinence was 9.5% in this group where the mean age was 54.9 years old. They found no difference in rates of fecal incontinence between nulliparous (11.3%), primiparous (9%), and multiparous (10.4%) women. Furthermore, they found that the difference in rates of fecal incontinence following vaginal delivery (9.3%) and cesarean delivery (6.6%) was not statistically significant.

The survey by McKinnie and colleagues[17] also reported on rates of anal and fecal incontinence. Thirteen percent of respondents reported bothersome anal incontinence. Again, the authors found no difference in fecal incontinence between women who delivered vaginally or by cesarean section. Similar to their findings for urinary incontinence, they found an increased risk of the development of fecal incontinence following pregnancy itself (OR 2.3). In the survey by Lukacz and colleagues[20] of women in the Kaiser Permenante system, the overall rate of anal incontinence was 17% and there was no difference regardless of parity or mode of delivery. The survey by Altman and colleagues[19] of Swedish women 10 years after their first vaginal or cesarean delivery assessed fecal incontinence through validated questionnaires. Fecal incontinence to loose stools was equal between the two groups at 6% and to solid stools at 2% and 2.5%, respectively. Similarly, Goldberg and colleagues[25] concluded cesarean section was not protective against the development of fecal incontinence.

A systematic review of obstetric factors associated with the occurrence of symptoms of anal incontinence in the first year postpartum was performed in 2008.[26] The review concluded that mode of delivery appeared to influence the occurrence of anal incontinence only when flatus was included in the definition. There were no statistical differences between the development of incontinence to solid or liquid stool in women undergoing vaginal delivery versus cesarean within the first year postpartum. The systematic review confirmed an association of forceps and fecal incontinence, finding that forceps doubled the risk compared with nonoperative vaginal deliveries.

As with urinary incontinence, there are data to suggest that labor itself, and not just mode of delivery, is associated with the development of anal incontinence. Fynes and colleagues[27] performed a prospective cohort study of 234 women in Ireland. The authors performed anorectal physiology studies with anal manometry and measurement of pudendal nerve terminal motor latency 6 weeks postpartum. They found that 29% of women who had a vaginal delivery had impaired terminal motor latency compared with 9% of women delivering by cesarean. Women delivered by cesarean late in labor, after 8 cm dilated, had prolonged motor latency and reduced levator muscle strength compared with those with cesareans performed in early labor. They concluded that cesarean delivery performed after cervical dilation of 8 cm failed to protect the anal sphincter mechanism.

THE EFFECT OF ROUTE OF DELIVERY ON SEXUAL FUNCTION

The effect of vaginal delivery on pelvic floor muscles and nerves has been theorized to have an adverse effect on short- and long-term sexual function. Nerve injury during vaginal delivery may lead to difficulty with sensation, arousal, or orgasm. Multiple studies have been performed to examine the effects of mode of delivery on sexual satisfaction in the postpartum year and have found no differences between sexual satisfaction and mode of delivery.[28,29] Gungor and colleagues[30] also found no difference in sexual satisfaction of males regardless of their partner's mode of delivery. The CAPS cohort was also queried in respect to sexual activity and sexual function at 6 months postpartum using validated questionnaires. Although women with deliveries complicated by anal sphincter lacerations were less likely to report sexual activity within the 6 months postpartum (88% versus 94%), there were no differences in sexual function scores.[11]

SUMMARY

This review of published literature suggests that although urinary and anal incontinence may be increased following vaginal delivery, pregnancy itself is likely to lead to some degree of pelvic floor dysfunction regardless of mode of delivery. Furthermore, the prevalence of urinary and anal incontinence equalizes at the approximate time of menopause. The duration of any protective effect afforded by a cesarean section on the pelvic floor may be variable depending on the age of the woman at time of delivery.

Although cesarean sections are the most common gynecologic surgery performed in the United States, they do not go without risk. The rates of abnormal placentation, bladder injury, and blood loss are positively correlated with the number of repeat cesareans performed. Counseling of pregnant women who are considering an elective cesarean delivery for the sole purpose of the prevention of urinary and fecal incontinence should reflect the current data:

- Most women do not develop urinary or fecal incontinence postpartum.
- Prelabor cesarean sections are associated with lower rates of urinary incontinence, at least in the short-term.
- The rates of urinary and fecal incontinence increase following any pregnancy, and eventually equalize with increasing age despite mode of delivery.

REFERENCES

1. MacDorman M, Menacker F, Declercq E. Cesarean birth in the United States: epidemiology, trends, and outcomes. Clin Perinatol 2008;35:293–307.
2. Viswanathan M, Visco A, Hartmann K, et al. Cesarean delivery on maternal request. Evidence report/technology assessment number 133. Rockville (MD): Agency for Healthcare Research and Quality; 2006.
3. American College of Obstetricians and Gynecologists. Cesarean delivery on maternal request. Committee Opinion Number 394. Obstet Gynecol 2007;110: 1501–4.
4. Minkoff H, Chervenak FA. Elective primary cesarean delivery. N Engl J Med 2003; 348(10):946–50.
5. Sultan A, Kamm M, Hudson C. Pudendal nerve damage during labour: prospective study before and after childbirth. Br J Obstet Gynaecol 1994;101(1):22–8.
6. Lee S, Park J. Follow-up evaluation of the effect of vaginal delivery on the pelvic floor. Dis Colon Rectum 2000;43(11):1550–5.
7. Snooks S, Swash M, Mathers S, et al. Effect of vaginal delivery on the pelvic floor: a 5-year follow-up. Br J Surg 1990;77(12):1358–60.
8. Hu T, Wagner T, Bentkover J, et al. Costs of urinary incontinence and overactive bladder in the United States: a comparative study. Urology 2004;63(3):461–5.
9. Rortveit G, Daltveit AK, Hannestad YS, et al. Urinary incontinence after vaginal delivery of cesarean section. N Engl J Med 2003;348(10):900–7.
10. Van Brummen HJ, Bruinse HW, van de Pol G, et al. The effect of vaginal and cesarean delivery on lower urinary tract symptoms: what makes the difference? Int Urogynecol J 2007;18:133–9.
11. Borello-France D, Burgio KL, Richter HE, et al. Fecal and urinary incontinence in primiparous women. Obstet Gynecol 2006;108(4):863–72.
12. Altman D, Ekstrom A, Forsgren C, et al. Symptoms of anal and urinary incontinence following cesarean section or spontaneous vaginal delivery. Am J Obstet Gynecol 2007;197:512e1–7.
13. Goldberg RP, Abramov Y, Botros S, et al. Delivery mode is a major environmental determinant of stress urinary incontinence: results of the Evanston-Northwestern Twin Sisters Study. Am J Obstet Gynecol 2005;193:2149–53.
14. Handa VL, Harvey L, Fox HE, et al. Parity and route of delivery: does cesarean delivery reduce bladder symptoms later in life? Am J Obstet Gynecol 2004; 191:463–9.

15. Connolly TJ, Litman HJ, Tennstedt SL, et al. The effect of mode of delivery, parity, and birth weight on risk of urinary incontinence. Int Urogynecol J 2007;18: 1033–42.

16. Buchsbaum GH, Chin M, Glantz C, et al. Prevalence of urinary incontinence and associated risk factors in a cohort of nuns. Am J Obstet Gynecol 2002;100:226–9.

17. McKinnie V, Swift SE, Wang W, et al. The effect of pregnancy and mode of delivery on the prevalence of urinary and fecal incontinence. Am J Obstet Gynecol 2005;193:512–8.

18. Groutz A, Rimon E, Peled S, et al. Cesarean section: does it really prevent the development of postpartum stress urinary incontinence? A prospective study of 363 women one year after their first delivery. Neurourol Urodyn 2004;23:2–6.

19. Altman D, Ekstrom A, Gustafsson C, et al. Risk of urinary incontinence after childbirth: a 10-year prospective cohort study. Obstet Gynecol 2006;108(4):873–8.

20. Lukacz ES, Lawrence JM, Contreras R, et al. Parity, mode of delivery, and pelvic floor disorders. Obstet Gynecol 2006;107(6):1253–60.

21. Press JZ, Klein MC, Kaczorowski J, et al. Does cesarean section reduce postpartum urinary incontinence? A systematic review. Birth 2007;34(3):228–37.

22. Zetterstrom J, Mellgren A, Jensen LL, et al. Effect of vaginal delivery on anal sphincter morphology and function. Dis Colon Rectum 1999;42(10):1253–60.

23. Zetterstrom JP, Lopez A, Anzen B, et al. Anal incontinence after vaginal delivery: a prospective study in primiparous women. Br J Obstet Gynaecol 1999;106: 324–30.

24. Fritel X, Ringa V, Varnoux N, et al. Mode of delivery and fecal incontinence at midlife: a study of 2640 women in the Gazel cohort. Obstet Gynecol 2007; 110(1):31–8.

25. Goldberg RP, Kwon C, Gandhi S, et al. Prevalence of anal incontinence among mothers of multiples and analysis of risk factors. Am J Obstet Gynecol 2003; 189:1627–30.

26. Pretlove SJ, Thompson PJ, Toozs-Hobson PM, et al. Does the mode of delivery predispose women to anal incontinence in the first year postpartum? A comparative systematic review. BJOG 2008;115:421–34.

27. Fynes M, Donnelly VS, O'Connell PR, et al. Cesarean delivery and anal sphincter injury. Obstet Gynecol 1998;92(4):496–500.

28. Woranitat W, Taneepanichskul S. Sexual function during the postpartum period. J Med Assoc Thai 2007;90(9):1744–8.

29. Botros SM, Abramov Y, Miller JR, et al. Effect of parity on sexual function: an identical twin study. Obstet Gynecol 2006;107(4):765–70.

30. Gungor S, Baser I, Ceyhan T, et al. Does mode of delivery affect sexual functioning of the man partner? J Sex Med 2008;5(1):155–63.

The Economics of Elective Cesarean Section

John A.F. Zupancic, MD, ScD[a,b,*]

KEYWORDS

- Cesarean section • Surgical procedures, elective
- Costs and cost analysis

The rate of cesarean section deliveries has increased markedly over the past decade and now constitutes almost one third of deliveries in the United States.[1] Although the reasons for this increase are multifactorial, it is notable that the frequency of such deliveries for mothers who have no indicated medical risk is also rising dramatically to 6.9% overall and 11.2% in primiparous mothers.[1–4] Four million deliveries occur annually in the United States,[5] and obstetric care has traditionally constituted a substantial portion of medical costs for young women, as well as being a major source of uncompensated care.[6] The economic implications of a large shift in the mode of delivery are, therefore, potentially important. This article reviews the relevant economic issues surrounding elective cesarean section and cesarean section at maternal request, summarizes the methodological quality and results of current literature on the topic, and presents recommendations for further study.

THE UNUSUAL CASE OF ELECTIVE DELIVERY

The annual health expenditure in the United States is approximately 2.2 trillion dollars or 16% of the gross domestic product.[7] Such a substantial investment is made with the intention of improving some aspect of the health of participants in the system. This estimate highlights that fact that the health care system does not restrict itself to offering therapies that save money. Interventions may have a net cost up to an acceptable level provided there is some benefit that accrues to patients or society. For this reason, economic studies are classified according to whether they examine only costs (cost analysis), or whether they simultaneously examine both costs and

[a] Division of Newborn Medicine, Harvard Medical School, 300 Longwood Avenue, Enders 9, Boston, MA, USA
[b] Department of Neonatology, Beth Israel Deaconess Medical Center, 330 Brookline Avenue, Rose Building Room 318, Boston, MA 02215, USA
* Department of Neonatology, Beth Israel Deaconess Medical Center, 330 Brookline Avenue, Rose Building Room 318, Boston, MA 02215, USA.
E-mail address: jzupanci@bidmc.harvard.edu

Clin Perinatol 35 (2008) 591–599
doi:10.1016/j.clp.2008.07.001
0095 5108/08/$ – see front matter © 2008 Elsevier Inc. All rights reserved.

effects (cost-effectiveness or cost-benefit analysis). Cost-effectiveness analyses are preferred because they provide information on whether an intervention saves money as well as whether it costs money but has an acceptable value for the money invested. The weighing of costs and effects is presented as a "cost-effectiveness ratio," which is the difference in the costs between cesarean section and vaginal delivery divided by the difference in outcomes.

The most important issue in understanding the economics of cesarean section on maternal request is whether there is, in fact, any benefit that accrues to the mother, infant, or society. If cesarean section on maternal request were indeed medically completely unnecessary (ie, without any benefits at all), any investment of resources would be economically wise only if either operative or vaginal delivery cost less. On the other hand, if mothers request an elective delivery to reduce risks, an investment in the intervention may be worthwhile if the costs are reasonable relative to the improved outcomes. The accounting of risks and benefits of alternative modes of delivery has been the subject of several articles in this series.[8-11] A National Institutes of Health State-of-the-Science Conference panel determined in a systematic review that moderate quality evidence was available linking cesarean section on maternal request with a decreased risk of maternal hemorrhage as well as increased neonatal respiratory morbidity, subsequent placenta previa or accreta, subsequent uterine rupture, and a longer maternal length of stay.[12,13] Weak evidence links elective cesarean section with a lower risk of neonatal encephalopathy, brachial plexus injury, and short-term (but not long-term) urinary incontinence. Each of these outcomes has potential economic implications that will be examined further herein.

Significant changes have occurred in the financing and delivery of obstetric care over the past 20 years. Moreover, the generalizability of health care information across international borders is of uncertain significance. To maintain relevance for the current system, this review concentrates on literature published since 1995 using North American data.

METHODOLOGICAL CONSIDERATIONS IN THE ECONOMICS LITERATURE FOR ELECTIVE CESAREAN SECTION

Before the studies referenced in this review are used in making policy decisions, it is important to understand their potential methodological limitations. **Table 1** presents characteristics of published studies and highlights some issues that might affect internal or external validity of the results reported.

Studies of costs may be biased by the same factors that plague studies of clinical outcomes. The traditional hierarchy of evidence applies equally to economics, that is, randomized controlled trials provide optimal protection from systematic bias by distributing factors that might affect outcome randomly between groups, whereas non-controlled studies provide the least protection. In the context of elective cesarean section, only one randomized controlled study has been published with economic outcomes, a study of elective cesarean section for breech presentation. The remainder of studies are retrospective cohort studies (with inherent risk for bias through case selection or incomplete or inaccurate data) or computer models known as decision analyses. The latter typically involve a large number of assumptions and the use of secondary literature and are also prone to bias.

Elective cesarean section is often undertaken to avoid uncommon risks such as neonatal neurologic injury or maternal hemorrhage. In addition to being important clinical outcomes, such adverse events may have important economic consequences. For example, one case of cerebral palsy will have lifetime costs that exceed the cost differences for several hundred deliveries.[14] For this reason, studies must be

Table 1
Study characteristics

Study	Location	Type	Cohort Size	Cost Categories	Time Horizon	Costs Versus Charges	Data Sources	Uncertainty
Bost[17]	Texas (community hospital)	Retrospective cohort	Not specified	Direct medical (excluded overhead, MD, NICU)	Discharge	Costs	Financial database	Not assessed
Allen[31]	Canada (provincial)	Retrospective cohort	CS: 859 SVD: 16,690	Direct medical (excluded overhead)	Discharge	Costs	Administrative database	Statistical
Kazandjian[27]	Maryland (three urban hospitals)	Retrospective cohort	VD: 860 (141 included) CS: 186	Direct medical	Discharge	Charges	Hospital chart	Statistical
Palencia[22]	Multinational	RCT	VD arm 511 CS arm: 514	Direct medical	6 Weeks postpartum	Costs	RCT data	Statistical
Traynor[19]	Chicago (single site)	Retrospective cohort	VD: 50 CS: 50	Direct medical (excluded NICU, MD)	Discharge	Charges	Financial database	Statistical
Clark[20]	22 Hospitals in four states	Decision analysis	Not applicable	Direct medical (excluded MD)	Long-run (not specified)	Costs	Financial database	Not assessed
Chung[18]	Stanford	Decision analysis	Not applicable	All	Lifetime	Costs	Financial database	Sensitivity analysis
Dimaio[21]	Florida (single site)	Retrospective cohort	TOL: 139 CS: 65	Direct medical (excluded MD)	Discharge	Costs	Medical record, financial database	Statistical
Mauldin[23]	South Carolina	Retrospective cohort	VD: 41 CS: 24	Direct medical (excluded MD)	Discharge	Charges	Medical record, financial database	Statistical

Abbreviations: CS, cesarean section; MD, medical doctor; NICU, neonatal intensive care unit; RCT, randomized controlled trial; TOL, trial of labor; VD, vaginal delivery.

powered to detect differences in these outcomes, both clinically and economically. As shown in **Table 2**, estimates of the cost of elective cesarean section are often based on studies with fewer than 100 patients, resulting in poor estimates of the cost implications of rare events.

Similarly, many adverse events may have cost implications that extend beyond the immediate peripartum period. For elective cesarean section, these implications include the long-term effects of injury to the infant such as neurologic events and brachial plexus palsy, as well as the potential need for operative delivery in future pregnancies for the mother. None of the studies followed actual patients past 6 weeks postpartum, although two decision analyses attempted to model such outcomes using data from secondary sources.

The choice of which costs to include is a critical decision in economic analyses. Categories include direct costs, which refer to those costs that can be assigned to individual patients. These costs include direct medical costs, such as hospital, drug, and physician fees, and direct nonmedical costs, such as the cost of parking or meals while receiving medical treatment. Overhead costs refer to costs that are shared between patients, such as heating or administrative costs for the hospital. Indirect or productivity costs are those related to decreased earning or work contribution by the patient or family during an illness or as a consequence of a chronic outcome. Because economic evaluations will be used to determine policy for a broad community, the ideal approach in economic analyses is to take a "societal perspective" in which one attempts to report all costs, regardless of the parties to whom they accrue. Individuals with particular interests, like the government or insurers, may then take a more restricted perspective. As shown in **Table 1**, all of the studies with the exception of one decision analysis omitted large cost categories, and none actually measured out-of-pocket expenses and work absences that might be of critical importance to patients. This approach mirrors the situation in neonatal cost studies more generally[15] but may affect the conclusions of economic evaluations comparing treatment modalities.

Regardless of the types of costs included, they must represent the actual cost of applying an intervention rather than charges for treatment.[16] In contrast to true costs, charges may reflect market conditions and demand for services, and may also include idiosyncratic attempts by the hospital provider to recoup costs from other aspects of its operation that cannot be directed elsewhere. Three of the nine studies of elective cesarean section actually report charges rather than costs; therefore, they should be viewed more critically.

Any study of patient-level data should report the degree of statistical uncertainty in the results. This uncertainty may be determined by traditional descriptive statistics or hypothesis testing, or by sensitivity analysis in which input parameters such as costs for a component of a therapy are varied through a range and the impact on the final results assessed. For elective cesarean section, most studies report using traditional statistical methods; two studies did not give any assessment of uncertainty.

ESTIMATES OF COSTS FOR ELECTIVE CESAREAN SECTION

This review did not retrieve any studies that specifically followed the economic outcomes of women who had requested cesarean section without medical indications. As a proxy for cesarean section on maternal request, several studies have followed patients who underwent cesarean section "electively" due to increased possible risk for adverse outcomes with a vaginal delivery. These situations included repeat cesarean section following a prior operative delivery, as compared with a trial of

Table 2
Cost estimates by delivery type for elective cesarean section

Study	Currency Date	Currency	Vaginal Delivery Spontaneous	Induction	Cesarean Section With Labor	Cesarean Section Without Labor	Comments
Bost[17]	Not specified, ?2001	US dollar	779	972	—	918	Induced VD estimate includes oxytocin and epidural; spontaneous VD estimate includes neither
Allen[31]	2004	US dollar	1340	—	2137	1532	Refer to text for long-run study results
Kazandjian[27]	Not specified ?2004	US dollar	17,624	—	13,805	—	NICU admission rate: 41% SVD, 22% CS; SVD included only top quartile by cost
Palencia[22]	2002	Canadian dollar	8042	—	7165	—	Estimates based on intention to treat; All estimates for breech VD
Traynor[19]	Not specified ?2003	US dollar	VBAC: 5289 No CS: 4685	—	8613 (failed TOL)	6785	Women with infants admitted to NICU excluded
Clark[20]	Not specified ?1996	US dollar	TOL: 2611	—	—	3042	Refer to text for long-run study results
Chung[18]	1999	US dollar	TOL: 4950	—	8414 (failed TOL)	7244	All estimates for TOL after previous cesarean
Dimaio[21]	1999	US dollar	VBAC: 4411	—	6272 (failed TCL)	5949	
Mauldin[23]	1996	US dollar	5890	—	—	7814	All pregnancies twin vertex/nonvertex VD by breech extraction of nonvertex twin

Abbreviations: CS, cesarean section; NICU, neonatal intensive care unit; SVD, spontaneous vaginal delivery; TOL, trial of labor; VBAC, vaginal birth after cesarean; VD, vaginal delivery.

labor;[17–21] twin or singleton breech presentation;[22,23] fetal macrosomia;[24,25] and low-risk nulliparous or unselected pregnancies.[26,27] Other studies of elective cesarean section for the avoidance of transmission of infectious illness were omitted because they may not be as generalizable.[28,29]

Cost estimates for cesarean section and vaginal delivery varied widely across studies. Similar results were reported in an earlier systematic review[30] and most likely result from the methodological differences detailed previously. For cesarean section without labor, cost estimates ranged from $918 to $7814.

When compared with uncomplicated vaginal delivery or a successful vaginal delivery after prior cesarean section, elective cesarean section is more expensive in most reported studies, with cost differences ranging from $139[17] to $2294.[18] Such differences probably most closely capture the cost implications of cesarean section on maternal request; however, comparison of elective cesarean section with a trial of labor may not yield cost savings, because a proportion of such trials lead to operative delivery, resulting in higher costs due to a longer duration of stay in labor and delivery, with its associated intensive personnel costs. In each case in which investigators reported cost estimates of cesarean section with labor and without labor, the latter were always higher.[18,19,21,31]

The restricted time horizon for all of the included studies likely results in an underestimate of costs for all types of deliveries due, in part, to the higher likelihood of repeat cesarean section. In a follow-up to the prior study of costs associated with initial delivery in a provincial database, Allen and colleagues[31] examined costs for each subsequent pregnancy. The cumulative cost through the third delivery was highest if the first delivery was by cesarean section with labor ($9524), with slightly lower estimates if the initial delivery was cesarean section without labor ($7213) or spontaneous vaginal delivery ($6425). Similarly, in a population-based Taiwanese study, elective cesarean section was followed by slightly higher expenditures for postpartum outpatient visits.[32]

Adverse events such as maternal hemorrhage are known to be associated with cesarean section but were seen rarely in the studies reviewed, because these studies did not have adequate power to detect uncommon events reliably. Such adverse consequences would be expected to increase the cost of cesarean section, but the amount of this increase is unknown. A more frequent adverse consequence of cesarean section may be prematurity resulting from incorrect dating of the pregnancy before scheduling of repeat section or from the fact that any elective scheduling will shift the mean delivery slightly earlier in gestation. Indeed, the frequency of late preterm birth has been increasing in concert with the increase in elective delivery.[33] The estimates for the costs associated with elective cesarean section were derived from studies that included only term infants. Prematurity is estimated to cost more than $26 billion annually in the United States, and much of this expenditure is for the care of late preterm infants.[15,34] The adoption of any intervention that increases the frequency of prematurity might have important and as yet unmeasured economic consequences.

Cost-Effectiveness Analyses

This review has thus far concentrated on determining whether there is a cost difference between elective cesarean section and vaginal delivery. Nevertheless, few medical interventions actually save money, and our society is willing to expend resources to improve health, provided that the expenditure has an acceptable health benefit. This balancing of costs and benefits is summarized using cost-effectiveness analyses in which both the costs and effects are typically presented in a single metric called the cost-effectiveness ratio. Unfortunately, few cost-effectiveness analyses have been performed for cesarean section. Culligan and colleagues[35] used decision analysis to compare standard care with a policy of routine ultrasound at 39 weeks followed by elective cesarean section for pregnancies with an estimated fetal weight above 4500 g. Their model yielded a reduction in anal incontinence and brachial plexus injury as well as reduced cost. The applicability of these results to maternal request cesarean section is unclear. Indeed, an earlier decision analysis that examined a similar intervention showed an unfavorable cost-effectiveness in women who did not have additional risk for macrosomia from diabetes mellitus;[25] therefore, it is unlikely that elective cesarean section would have appealing cost-effectiveness in an unselected population.

THE ECONOMICS OF MATERNAL PREFERENCE

Despite conflicting evidence, higher costs, and the potential risks of cesarean section without medical indication, some women may still want to undertake the procedure because of anxiety or a desire to reduce certain maternal and neonatal outcomes. In economic terms, these women might place a higher value on perceived benefits and a lower value on perceived risks. Such weighting of preferences can be quantified through patient interview and expressed as a "utility" or "willingness to pay."[36,37] Such preferences might help to prioritize policy regarding which interventions to offer. To date, no studies appear to have assessed maternal preferences for elective cesarean section in this manner.

SUMMARY

The frequency of cesarean section without medical indication, and in particular cesarean section on maternal request, appears to be increasing in the United States. The cost implications of such a policy are unclear and will depend largely on whether future studies establish that the practice has clinical benefits. The economic literature to date is limited to elective cesarean section rather than maternal request delivery. Cesarean section without labor does appear to be more expensive than uncomplicated vaginal delivery, but studies are seriously methodologically flawed, with few randomized trials, inadequate power, the omission of important types of costs including those accruing to patients, and the failure to report costs and effects together.

The economic outcomes associated with elective cesarean section are critically important. In the absence of a rigorously demonstrated benefit, any increased expenditure on an intervention will reduce the resources that are available for other medically necessary care. Given the high frequency of underinsured and vulnerable individuals in this population, the opportunity cost may very well be worse health overall.

It is not impossible to address the deficiencies in content and methodology outlined in this review. High-quality economic evaluations with a societal perspective should be undertaken prospectively alongside any large clinical studies so that the results are available to decision makers and clinicians as policy is being planned.

REFERENCES

1. Macdorman MF, Menacker F, Declercq E. Cesarean birth in the United States: epidemiology, trends, and outcomes. Clin Perinatol 2008;35:293–307.
2. Declercq E, Menacker F, MacDorman M. Rise in "no indicated risk" primary caesareans in the United States, 1991–2001: cross sectional analysis. BMJ 2005;330: 71–2.

3. Bailit JL, Love TE, Mercer B. Rising cesarean rates: are patients sicker? Am J Obstet Gynecol 2004;191:800–3.
4. Gregory KD, Korst LM, Gornbein JA, et al. Using administrative data to identify indications for elective primary cesarean delivery. Health Serv Res 2002;37: 1387–401.
5. Martin JA, Kung HC, Mathews TJ, et al. Annual summary of vital statistics: 2006. Pediatrics 2008;121:788–801.
6. Long SH, Marquis MS, Harrison ER. The costs and financing of perinatal care in the United States. Am J Public Health 1994;84:1473–8.
7. Poisal JA, Truffer C, Smith S, et al. Health spending projections through 2016: modest changes obscure part D's impact. Health Aff (Millwood) 2007;26: w242–53.
8. Signore C, Klebanoff M. Neonatal morbidity and mortality after elective cesarean delivery. Clin Perinatol 2008;35:361–71.
9. Ramachandrappa A, Jain L. Elective cesarean section: its impact on neonatal respiratory outcome. Clin Perinatol 2008;35:373–93.
10. Bettegowda VR, Dias T, Davidoff MJ, et al. The relationship between cesarean delivery and gestational age among US singleton births. Clin Perinatol 2008;35: 309–23.
11. Adams-Chapman I. Long-term neurologic outcome of infants born by cesarean section. Clin Perinatol 2008;35:437–54.
12. American College of Obstetricians and Gynecologists. ACOG Committee Opinion No. 394, December 2007. Cesarean delivery on maternal request. Obstet Gynecol 2007;110:1501.
13. NIH State-of-the-Science Conference Statement on cesarean delivery on maternal request. NIH Consens State Sci Statements 2006;23:1–29.
14. US Department of Health and Human Services, Centers for Disease Control and Prevention. Economic costs associated with mental retardation, cerebral palsy, hearing loss, and vision impairment–United States, 2003. MMWR Morb Mortal Wkly Rep 2004;53(3):57–9.
15. Zupancic JAF. A systematic review of costs associated with preterm birth. In: Behrman R, Stith-Butler A, editors. Preterm birth: causes, consequences and prevention. Washington, DC: The National Academies Press; 2006.
16. Finkler SA. The distinction between cost and charges. Ann Intern Med 1982;96: 102–9.
17. Bost BW. Cesarean delivery on demand: what will it cost? Am J Obstet Gynecol 2003;188:1418–21.
18. Chung A, Macario A, El-Sayed YY, et al. Cost-effectiveness of a trial of labor after previous cesarean. Obstet Gynecol 2001;97:932–41.
19. Traynor JD, Peaceman AM. Maternal hospital charges associated with trial of labor versus elective repeat cesarean section. Birth 1998;25:81–4.
20. Clark SL, Scott JR, Porter TF, et al. Is vaginal birth after cesarean less expensive than repeat cesarean delivery? Am J Obstet Gynecol 2000;182:599–602.
21. DiMaio H, Edwards RK, Euliano TY, et al. Vaginal birth after cesarean delivery: an historic cohort cost analysis. Am J Obstet Gynecol 2002;186:890–2.
22. Palencia R, Gafni A, Hannah ME, et al. The costs of planned cesarean versus planned vaginal birth in the term breech trial. CMAJ 2006;174:1109–13.
23. Mauldin JG, Mauldin PD, Feng TI, et al. Determining the clinical efficacy and cost savings of successful external cephalic version. Am J Obstet Gynecol 1996;175: 1639–44.

24. Herbst MA. Treatment of suspected fetal macrosomia: a cost-effectiveness analysis. Am J Obstet Gynecol 2005;193(3 Pt 2):1035–9.
25. Rouse DJ, Owen J, Goldenberg RL, et al. The effectiveness and costs of elective cesarean delivery for fetal macrosomia diagnosed by ultrasound. JAMA 1996; 276:1480–6.
26. Allen VM, O'Connell CM, Baskett TF. Cumulative economic implications of initial method of delivery. Obstet Gynecol 2006;108(3 Pt 1):549–55.
27. Kazandjian VA, Chaulk CP, Ogunbo S, et al. Does a cesarean section delivery always cost more than a vaginal delivery? J Eval Clin Pract 2007;13(1):16–20.
28. Mrus JM, Goldie SJ, Weinstein MC, et al. The cost-effectiveness of elective cesarean delivery for HIV-infected women with detectable HIV RNA during pregnancy. AIDS 2000;14:2543–52.
29. Chen KT, Sell RL, Tuomala RE. Cost-effectiveness of elective cesarean delivery in human immunodeficiency virus-infected women (1). Obstet Gynecol 2001;97(2): 161–8.
30. Henderson J, McCandlish R, Kumiega L, et al. Systematic review of economic aspects of alternative modes of delivery. BJOG 2001;108:149–57.
31. Allen VM, O'Connell CM, Farrell SA, et al. Economic implications of method of delivery. Am J Obstet Gynecol 2005;193:192–7.
32. Liu TC, Chen CS, Lin HC. Does elective caesarean section increase utilization of postpartum maternal medical care? Med Care 2008;46:440–3.
33. Fuchs K, Gyamfi C. The influence of obstetric practices on late prematurity. Clin Perinatol 2008;35:343–60.
34. Waitzman NJ, Rogowski J. Societal costs of preterm birth. In: Behrman R, Stith-Butler A, editors. Preterm birth: causes, consequences and prevention. Washington, DC: The National Academies Press; 2006. p. 398–429.
35. Culligan PJ, Myers JA, Goldberg RP, et al. Elective cesarean section to prevent anal incontinence and brachial plexus injuries associated with macrosomia: a decision analysis. Int Urogynecol J Pelvic Floor Dysfunct 2005;16:19–28.
36. Petrou S, Henderson J. Preference-based approaches to measuring the benefits of perinatal care. Birth 2003;30:217–26.
37. Henderson J, Petrou S. The economic case for planned cesarean section for breech presentation at term. CMAJ 2006;174:1118–9.

Index

Note: Page numbers of article titles are in **boldface** type.

Clin Perinatol 35 (2008) 601–608
doi:10.1016/S0095-5108(08)00072-9   perinalology.theclinics.com
0095-5108/08/$ – see front matter © 2008 Elsevier Inc. All rights reserved.

Moving?

Make sure your subscription moves with you!

To notify us of your new address, find your **Clinics Account Number** (located on your mailing label above your name), and contact customer service at:

E-mail: elspcs@elsevier.com

800-654-2452 (subscribers in the U.S. & Canada)
1-407-563-6020 (subscribers outside of the U.S. & Canada)

Fax number: 407-363-9661

Elsevier Periodicals Customer Service
6277 Sea Harbor Drive
Orlando, FL 32887-4800

*To ensure uninterrupted delivery of your subscription, please notify us at least 4 weeks in advance of move.